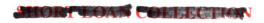
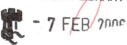

An Atlas of
EAR, NOSE AND THROAT
DISORDERS

THE ENCYCLOPEDIA OF VISUAL MEDICINE SERIES

An Atlas of
EAR, NOSE AND
THROAT DISORDERS

A. Julianna Gulya, MD, FACS

Clinical Professor of Surgery
(Otolaryngology–Head and Neck Surgery)
The George Washington University
Washington, DC

Chief, Clinical Trials Branch,
National Institute on Deafness and Other Communication Disorders (NIDCD)

and

William R. Wilson, MD, FACS

Professor of Surgery
(Otolaryngology–Head and Neck Surgery)
Chief of the Division of Otolaryngology–Head and Neck Surgery
The George Washington University
Washington, DC

The Parthenon Publishing Group
International Publishers in Medicine, Science & Technology

NEW YORK   LONDON

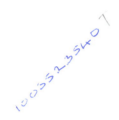

Library of Congress Cataloging-in-Publication Data

Gulya, Aina J.
    An atlas of ear, nose, and throat disorders / A. Julianna Gulya and
William R. Wilson.
        p. cm. -- (Encyclopedia of visual medicine series)
    Includes index.
    ISBN 1-85070-937-8 (alk. paper)
        I. Otolaryngology -- Atlases. I. Title. II. Series. III. Wilson, William R.
    [DNLM: I. Otorhinolaryngologic Diseases--Atlases. WV 17 G973a1999]
    RF46.5 .G84 1999
    617.5'1 21--dc21

                                                            99-040838

Published in the USA by
The Parthenon Publishing Group Inc.
One Blue Hill Plaza
PO Box 1564, Pearl River
New York 10965, USA

Published in the UK and Europe by
The Parthenon Publishing Group Limited
Casterton Hall, Carnforth
Lancs., LA6 2LA, UK

British Library Cataloguing in Publication Data

An atlas of ear, nose and throat disorders. - (The encyclopedia of visual
    medicine series)
    I. Otolaryngology
    I. Gulya, A. Julianna (Aina Julianna) II. Wilson, William R.
    617.5'1
    ISBN 1-85070-937-8

Printed and bound in Spain
by T.G. Hostench, S.A.

Contents

Preface

It is hoped that this Atlas will provide the active clinician with a useful reference and guide to the disorders of the ear, nose and throat – and also that it may encourage and help those currently planning to specialize in the field of otolaryngology.

The illustrations included in this atlas were culled from thousands of photographs (largely derived from the authors' practices), and constitute those which illustrate important otolaryngological concepts and /or disorders with the highest possible quality.

Of course, it was not the intention of the authors to provide an in-depth and comprehensive textbook of otolaryngological disorders and diseases since a number of such textbooks are already available. Rather, the objective of this Atlas is to illustrate with as much clarity as possible a wide range of conditions where proper visual perception is essential for correct clinical diagnosis.

We thank Drs Eiji and Ken Yanagisawa, who so graciously provided Figures 10, 11 and 23, and Dr Steven Bielomazwicz, who so kindly contributed Chapter 5 on the normal structure, function and disorders of the human larynx.

A. J. Gulya
W. R. Wilson

Section 1 A Review of Ear, Nose and Throat Disorders

Ear

Anatomy

The ear is divided into three compartments: external; middle; and inner. The external ear consists of the pinna (or auricle), external auditory canal and tympanic membrane, and serves as a funnel to transmit sound, traveling in the form of alternating waves of compressed and rarefied air, to the middle ear. The middle ear contains three ossicles in a sequential chain, namely, the malleus, incus and stapes, which conduct sound across the tympanic cavity to the organ of hearing in the inner ear, the cochlea. The middle ear has two muscles: the tensor tympani, which attaches to the malleus; and the stapedius, which is attached to the stapes and modulates sound transmission. The footplate of the stapes occupies the oval window. The piston-like action of the stapes transmits sound energy to the cochlea.

The tympanic cavity is divided into three sections, according to the relationship to the margins of the tympanic membrane: the epitympanum (or attic) lies above; the hypotympanum below; and the mesotympanum in between the two. The eustachian tube is an anteroinferior extension of the tympanic cavity and extends to the posterior aspect of the nasopharynx.

The inner ear comprises the cochlea and labyrinth. The cochlea is a snail-shell-shaped structure containing three fluid-filled compartments: the scala tympani; scala vestibuli; and scala media, which houses the organ of Corti. The cochlea abuts the tympanic cavity at the membrane of the round window. The labyrinth consists of three semicircular canals (lateral, superior and inferior), two otolithic organs (the utricle and saccule) involved in the sense of balance and the vestibule. The cochlear, superior and inferior vestibular, and facial nerves traverse the internal auditory canal, located at the medial aspect of the inner ear.

The mastoid bone is located posterior and deep to the external auditory canal, from which it is separated by the posterior wall of the canal. The mastoid consists of irregularly shaped air-filled cells made up of thin, mucosa-lined, septa of bone. This air-cell system is continuous with the tympanic cavity at the level of the attic, and runs through the antrum and aditus ad antrum.

The facial nerve (cranial nerve VII) traverses the internal auditory canal, middle ear and mastoid in its intraosseous course to exit near the tip of mastoid at the stylomastoid foramen.

The internal carotid artery courses immediately anterior to the cochlea as it enters the cranial cavity. The sigmoid sinus runs in the posteromedial aspect of mastoid and drains venous blood from the transverse sinus to the internal jugular vein.

Physiology

The primary functions of the ear are hearing and balance. Because the cochlea, the organ of hearing in the inner ear, is a fluid-filled organ, sound waves that have been transmitted across the external auditory canal and ossicular chain undergo a transition from airborne vibrations to a fluid-displacement wave at the interface of the stapes and oval window. To compensate for the loss of sound intensity [approximately 30 decibels (dB)] as a result of this transition, the middle ear has an impedance-matching mechanism, or functional lever, consisting of the tympanic membrane and ossicular chain.

The fluid displacement initiated in the cochlea by displacement of the stapes travels from the base towards the apex and, as it travels, causes in turn a displacement of the basilar membrane on which the organ of Corti is located. The organ of Corti describes the system of outer and inner hair cells, their supporting cells and nerve endings, and the tectorial membrane, which blankets the hair cells and in which are embedded the cilia (hairs) of the hair cells.

The point of maximum displacement is specific for varying frequencies of sound; it is located at the base for high-frequency sounds, and moves progressively towards the apex for low-frequency sounds. Displacement of the basilar membrane also displaces the hair cells, resulting in a shearing motion of the hairs in relation to their cells, and an ion flow through the hair cells which activates their associated nerve endings. This excitatory activity is carried through the primary auditory neurons in the modiolus of the cochlea to higher auditory centers by the cochlear nerve, resulting in the perception of sound. Throughout this process, the tonotopic, or frequency-specific, arrangement is maintained.

Diagnostic evaluation

Physical examination

Examination of the ear begins with appraisal of the external ear for normal anatomy, then proceeds with otoscopy to inspect the external auditory canal and tympanic membrane. In examining the tympanic membrane, it is important to note the color and translucency of the normal drum. Key landmarks include the handle and lateral process of the malleus, and it is especially important to examine the area above the lateral process (Schrapnell's membrane) covering the attic. Pneumatic otoscopy allows assessment of the mobility of the tympanic membrane and the malleus.

Tuning fork testing is performed minimally with a 512 Hz fork. In the Weber test, the vibrating fork is placed firmly on the patient's forehead. Perceived sound lateralizing to the poorer-hearing ear indicates a conductive hearing loss in that ear whereas lateralization to the better-hearing ear is suggestive of a severe sensorineural hearing loss in the opposite ear. With the Rinne test, the vibrating fork is placed first on the bone of mastoid and then in front of the ear canal of the tested ear. Normally, the sound of the fork is perceived as being louder when placed in front of the ear canal ('positive' Rinne). In conductive hearing loss, the fork is perceived as being louder when placed on the mastoid bone ('negative' Rinne). If the fork is perceived in the non-test ear, a severe sensorineural hearing loss in the test ear should be suspected.

Diagnostic testing

The functional integrity of the auditory system is usually assessed by an audiogram (Figure 1, page 33), which includes pure-tone air and bone conduction testing, speech audiometry and impedance audiometry (Figure 2, page 33).

Pure-tone testing is usually carried out using 250–8000 Hz and, for air-conduction testing, the sounds are delivered through earphones to the test ear with masking, or interference noise, used as necessary to isolate the non-test ear. Air-conduction testing uses the same pathway as environmental sound, and evaluates the integrity of the conductive mechanism of the ear as well as cochlear function.

In bone-conduction testing, the pure-tone vibration is applied directly to the skull to directly stimulate the cochlea and bypass the conductive apparatus. By assessing air and bone thresholds – that is, the loudness required of the sound to be perceived for each modality – it is possible to determine whether hearing is normal or abnormal and whether hearing loss is due to a problem in the conductive mechanism (conductive hearing loss), dysfunction in the cochlea or cochlear nerve (sensorineural hearing loss) or dysfunction of both (mixed hearing loss).

A pure-tone average (PTA), the average of the thresholds obtained with air-conduction testing at 500, 1000 and 2000 Hz, is calculated (see Figure 1). Speech audiometry establishes a speech reception threshold (SRT), which is the level of loudness at which specific two-syllable words, balanced for equal emphasis on both syllables, are identified correctly 50% of the time.

Speech-discrimination testing uses the same type of two-syllable words delivered at 40 dB over the measured SRT, and records the percent of correctly identified words, which is the speech discrimination score (SDS). A poorer SDS than expected from the PTA should raise suspicion of a retrocochlear hearing loss, which involves structures medial to the cochlea, in particular, the cochlear nerve. With increasing loudness of presentation, the SDS generally improves and levels off whereas a steep dive in SDS is suggestive of a retrocochlear disorder.

Tympanometry measures the static volume of the ear canal, compliance of the middle ear and the stapedius reflex, using a carefully fitted ear plug in the test ear. A static volume measurement that is larger than expected suggests an unseen tympanic membrane perforation, although a mastoidectomy from the canal wall downwards also gives a large volume reading.

Compliance of the middle ear is assessed by applying positive and negative pressure (see Figure 2). Three types of compliance curves are recognized – A, B and C. The A curve peaks at 0 mm H$_2$O, indicating no pressure differential between the middle ear and the external environment, as expected in an ear with normal eustachian tube function. AS

indicates a 'stiff' middle ear system, as found in otosclerosis, whereas AD suggests ossicular discontinuity. The B curve suggests the presence of middle ear fluid, and the C curve indicates possible eustachian tube dysfunction with its consequential negative middle ear pressure.

Special testing

The auditory brain-stem response (ABR; Figure 3, page 34) measures the activity of the auditory system from the nerve endings in the cochlea through the central auditory structures as stimulated by sound. Normally, a series of five waves – I through V – is distinguishable, with a specific temporal relationship to the instigating sound and in relation to each other. ABR testing is useful in the detection of retrocochlear function and is also used in infant hearing screening, as no subject cooperation is required.

Electrocochleography (ECoG) is a test of the fluid-balance status of the inner ear. Normally, there are two deflections – the summating potential (SP) and the action potential (AP) – seen in sequence early after a sound stimulus. The SP-to-AP amplitude ratio is usually in the range of 50%; if it exceeds this value, the diagnosis of endolymphatic hydrops (overaccumulation of endolymph occupying the scala media, as seen in Meniere's disease) is suggested.

Otoacoustic emissions (OAEs) are a relatively new test of auditory function. The cochlear hair cells produce sound, both spontaneously and in response to sound, which is recorded in the external auditory canal to yield a measure of the functional integrity of the hair cells. OAEs are currently used in the screening of newborn hearing as well as in other auditory testing situations where patient cooperation is not possible.

Balance, or vestibular, testing is accomplished by electronystagmography (ENG), in which electrodes are placed above and lateral to the eyes to record eye movements by taking advantage of the natural electric dipole of the eyes. A series of tracking and positioning tests are performed as well as bithermal caloric testing of each ear. Caloric testing allows detection of hypofunction of one labyrinth in comparison to the other, whereas assessment of the tracking and positioning tests may provide evidence of specific labyrinthine dysfunction or disorders of the central nervous system.

Other tests of balance, such as posturography and sinusoidal harmonic acceleration, may be carried out for more specialized assessment of the vestibular system.

Imaging

Although plane X-rays of the ear may occasionally be helpful, for detailed visualization of the extent of middle ear and mastoid disease, a special computed tomography (CT) scan – temporal bone CT (see Figure 32, page 45) – is preferable. Ideally, serial sections 1–2 mm in thickness are obtained in both the axial and coronal planes with a bone-imaging algorithm. Usually, a review of the brain is also performed to seek out potential intracranial complications of ear disease.

Magnetic resonance imaging (MRI; see Figure 42, page 49), is able to provide outstanding images of soft tissue structures such as the brain but, at present, cannot reveal bony structures or bone erosion. Thus, its utility in the management of otological disease is in the delineation of associated brain complications such as cerebral abscess or herniation, and in the diagnosis of intracranial disorders such as acoustic neuromas (vestibular schwannomas).

Disorders

The more common disorders of the ear are shown in Figures 4–42 (see pages 35–49).

Nose

Anatomy and physiology

The nose has cosmetic, respiratory and olfactory functions. The cosmetically important external nose serves as a framework for the uppermost portion of the airways, and consists of bone and cartilage draped with skin and subcutaneous tissue. The internal nose is divided into two nasal cavities by a bony and cartilaginous nasal septum positioned in the midline.

The anterior apertures (nares or nostrils) open into the associated vestibules and are lined by squamous epithelium with standard skin adnexa. The remainder of the nasal cavity, except for the olfactory epithelium in the superior one-third of the cavity, is lined by pseudostratified ciliated columnar (respiratory) epithelium, which extends to the associated paranasal sinuses.

The lateral walls of the nasal cavities are subdivided by three turbinate bones – superior, middle and inferior – each with its associated meatus to provide drainage for the nasolacrimal duct and paranasal sinuses. The posterior apertures of the nasal cavity are the choanae, which open into the nasopharynx.

The subcutaneous tissue of the turbinate bones is highly vascular and anatomically reminiscent of erectile tissue. This tissue has an important role in the temperature regulatory function (of inspired air) of the nose. In addition, the mucociliary blanket of the respiratory epithelium serves as a filter to eliminate particulate debris from inspired air.

The midline septum is highly vascularized, particularly at its anteroinferior aspect (Little's area), the site of a vascular plexus which is often implicated in epistaxis. Also implicated in epistaxis are the anterior and posterior ethmoidal, and internal maxillary arteries.

Diagnostic evaluation

Physical examination

Nasal examination begins with inspection of the external nose with palpation as indicated, for example, in cases of trauma. Use of a nasal speculum to open the nasal vestibule provides a view of the anterior nasal cavity. Application of a topical vasoconstrictor, such as phenylephrine (Neo-Synephrine™) or oxymetazoline hydrochloride, shrinks the mucosal lining, resulting in improved visualization of the posterior and superior aspects of the nasal cavity. Rigid and flexible nasal endoscopy facilitate more detailed examination of the nose posteriorly into the nasopharynx.

Diagnostic testing

Standard Gram's staining of the nasal discharge, which may be performed in the office, is helpful in distinguishing between infectious and allergic (characterized by the presence of eosinophils) etiologies.

Imaging

Plane X-rays of the nose, especially in a lateral view, are helpful in delineating displaced fractures in cases of nasal trauma. CT and MRI may be useful in determining the extent of nasal, sinus and nasopharyngeal disease.

Special testing

Olfaction is readily assessed by commercially available 'scratch-and-sniff' kits.

Disorders

Disorders of the nose are illustrated in Figures 43–55 (see pages 49–53).

Paranasal sinuses

Anatomy and physiology

The paranasal sinuses develop as evaginations of the nasal cavity into the bones of the skull and are lined by the same respiratory epithelium. There are four pairs of sinuses: the frontal lie above the root of the nose and the orbits; the ethmoid are medial to the orbit; the maxillary are associated with the maxilla; and the sphenoid is located below the sella turcica.

The sinuses impart resonance characteristics to the voice and also reduce the weight of the skull. As with the mastoid bone, however, development of the sinuses demonstrates considerable inter-individual variability, especially the frontal sinuses, which may be underdeveloped or completely absent.

The drainage route for the mucociliary circulation of the sinuses is through their ostia into the nasal cavity. Accordingly, inflammatory conditions of the nose may cause reflex edema and obstruction of the ostia, leading to sinus infection.

Diagnostic evaluation

Physical examination

Examination for sinus disease is incorporated into the nasal and nasopharyngeal examinations, and is supplemented by percussion of the sinuses ('tap tenderness') and perhaps transillumination.

Imaging

Radiological techniques are of primary importance in the diagnosis and management of sinus disorders; these include plane X-rays, CT and, to a lesser extent, MRI. Some institutions offer a 'sinus screening' CT that reduces both the cost and exposure to radiation compared with a full CT scan, but still provides adequate imaging of the sinuses.

Disorders

Disorders of the paranasal sinuses are shown in Figures 56–64 (see pages 53–55).

Oral cavity and pharynx

Anatomy and physiology

The major structures of the oral cavity are the lips, teeth, tongue and palate (hard and soft). The oral cavity is involved in the initial processing of the food bolus, respiration and speech production. The openings of the major salivary glands, or puncta, are located in the oral cavity, specifically, in the floor of the mouth (submandibular glands) and in the cheeks opposite the second molar (parotid glands).

The pharynx is fundamentally a muscular column comprising superior, middle and inferior constrictor muscles. It is divided into three compartments: nasopharynx superiorly; oropharynx; and hypopharynx inferiorly. The adenoids are associated with the nasopharynx whereas the palatine tonsils are part of the oropharynx. The pharynx is involved in respiration and deglutition. The immunological activity of the pharynx emanates from the lymphoid elements of Waldeyer's ring, primarily the palatine tonsils, adenoids and lingual tonsils.

Diagnostic evaluation

Physical examination

Examination of the oral cavity and pharynx begins with inspection, and is extended by the use of indirect mirror examination or direct examination *via* flexible or rigid endoscopes. Bimanual palpation is especially helpful in the evaluation of the floor of the mouth and base of the tongue.

Imaging

Plane films are obtained as described for the paranasal sinuses (see page 18), but CT and MRI, both with the addition of contrast media, are usually more helpful in detecting and delineating the extent of disease in this area.

Special studies

The modified barium swallow, or videofluoroscopy, is a special form of the more familiar barium swallow and is especially useful in the evaluation of dysphagia. The modified barium swallow adds digital analysis of the video images derived from fluoroscopic studies, thereby allowing finer measurements and measuring techniques in the study of normal swallowing and the pathophysiology of abnormal swallowing. Videofluoroscopy permits examination of the oropharyngeal aspects of swallowing, such as bolus transit time, and duration of airway entry closure and cricopharyngeal opening, and their temporal interrelationships.

Disorders

Disorders of the oral cavity and pharynx are illustrated in Figures 65–101 (see pages 55–65).

Larynx
by Steven Bielomazwicz

Anatomy

The larynx comprises an intricate set of neuro-muscular units attached to a cartilaginous skeleton. The most important of these units are the cricoid, thyroid and arytenoid cartilages. The cricoid cartilage is the signet ring-shaped structure attached to the trachea which provides a solid foundation for the remainder of the larynx. The paired arytenoid cartilages rest on the posterosuperior surface of the cricoid cartilage, and move anteriorly and medially to effect glottal closure. The thyroid cartilage serves to protect and support the larynx.

The vocal ligaments, which attach to the vocal processes of the arytenoid cartilages and insert on the posterior surface of the thyroid cartilage, are the foundation of the superficial mucosal structures called the vocal folds. Each vocal fold is a multi-layered structure consisting of a body, a cover and a transition zone. The body is composed of the thyroarytenoid muscle and vocal ligament; the transition zone comprises the intermediate and deep layers of the lamina propria of the vocal ligament; and the epithelium and superficial layer of the lamina propria constitute the cover.

The adducting (glottal-closing) intrinsic muscles of the larynx are the thyroarytenoid, lateral cricoarytenoid and interarytenoid muscles. These are innervated by the recurrent laryngeal nerve (RLN), which also innervates the primary abducting muscle of the larynx, the posterior cricoarytenoid muscle. Motor input to the cricothyroid muscles and sensation in the supraglottic larynx are supplied by the external branch of the superior laryngeal nerve (SLN).

Physiology

The larynx has three primary functions: airway maintenance; prevention of aspiration; and voice production. The role of airway maintenance relies primarily on the structural and functional integrity of the larynx. The cricoid cartilage, which is the only complete ring, is the keystone of the architectural framework and serves to link the larynx to the trachea.

Prevention of aspiration into the lower airway is a complex function, requiring intact and co-ordinated sensory input to, and motor control of, both the larynx and pharynx. On swallowing, the larynx is elevated, thereby facilitating closure of the upper airway by the epiglottis complemented by adduction of the vocal folds. At the same time, the cricopharyngeal muscle opens, thus directing the food bolus away from the airway and into the esophagus.

Voice production is the third complex function of the larynx. Speech is produced by controlled exhalation across the adducting vocal folds, thereby causing the vocal fold mucosa to vibrate. Pitch is determined by the tension and stiffness of the vocal fold mucosa, volume by the rate of airflow, and clarity according to the symmetry of the vocal fold vibration pattern and the completeness of vocal fold closure.

Diagnostic evaluation

Physical examination

Evaluation of the larynx may be carried out with a mirror, a fiberoptic nasal endoscope or a rigid oral endoscope. Examination by mirror requires the least equipment and gives the skilled clinician a good assessment of the larynx with minimal optical distortion. However, the procedure is not well tolerated by individuals who have a sensitive gag reflex, and does not permit slow-motion assessment.

Fiberoptic endoscopic examination of the larynx is easily performed in the clinic by passing the endoscope through the topically anesthetized and decongested nose. Most patients find the examination comfortable. A wide range of voicing tasks may be assessed, including singing and whistling. The examination may be recorded by a closed-circuit camera, and a videocassette recording allows subsequent review with the patient. Use of a stroboscopic light source creates the illusion of slowing of the vocal fold vibration pattern to permit assessment of the subtle abnormalities of wave formation. Unfortunately, the equipment is expensive, and considerable skill is required to perform an adequate examination. Some image distortion is also inevitable.

A rigid oral endoscope, placed on the base of the tongue, provides a picture with excellent detail and a nearly flat field of view. The endoscope may be used with either straight or stroboscopic light. The examination may be videorecorded onto tape for later review. However, the range of voicing tasks is somewhat limited as the endoscope is placed between the lips and rests on the tongue.

Disorders

Disorders of the larynx are shown in Figures 102–117 (see pages 65–70).

Section II Ear, Nose and Throat Disorders Illustrated

List of illustrations

Figure 112

Rigid endoscopy showing generalized erythema (arrowed) of the larynx and pharynx due to gastroesophageal reflux

Figure 113

Rigid endoscopy showing granulomas on the body of the arytenoid cartilage due to gastro-esophageal reflux

Figure 114

Rigid endoscopy showing bowed vocal folds

Figure 115

Rigid endoscopy showing early laryngeal (glottic) squamous cell carcinoma

Figure 116

Rigid endoscopy showing advanced glottic squamous cell carcinoma

Figure 117

Rigid endoscopy showing supraglottic carcinoma (arrowed)

EAR

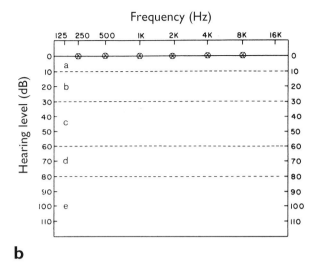

Figure 1 (a) Symbols commonly used in behavioral audiometry, and (b) audiogram showing normal hearing bilaterally. The a zone indicates the normal hearing range whereas zones b–e indicate mild, moderate, severe, and profound hearing losses, respectively. Reproduced with permission, from Wilson & Nadol Jr. *Quick Reference to Ear, Nose, and Throat Disorders*. Philadelphia: JB Lippincott, 1983

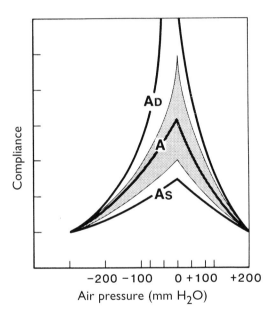
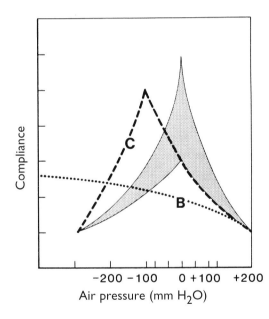

Figure 2 Middle ear compliance as measured by tympanometry. The A curve peaks at 0 mm H$_2$O, indicating no pressure differential between the middle ear and external environment (normal eustachian tube function). The AS curve indicates a 'stiff' middle ear system (as in otosclerosis), and the AD curve suggests ossicular discontinuity. The B curve suggests the presence of middle ear fluid whereas the C curve implies eustachian tube dysfunction with its consequent negative middle ear pressure. Reproduced with permission, from Wilson & Nadol Jr. *Quick Reference to Ear, Nose, and Throat Disorders*. Philadelphia: JB Lippincott, 1983

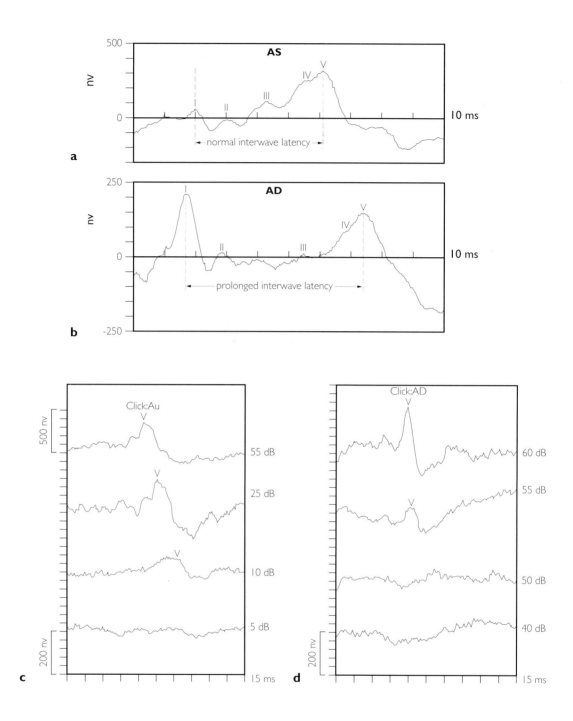

Figure 3 Tracings showing a normal auditory brain-stem response (ABR; a). All five waves are present, and occur at the expected time (latency) after the eliciting sound stimulus and at the expected intervals in relation to each other (interwave latency). In an ABR pattern suggestive of vestibular schwannoma (b), wave V is delayed in onset relative to time 0 (sound stimulus), and the interwave latency is prolonged. ABR tracings are also used to determine auditory thresholds. A wave V distinguishable at 10 dB is normal (c) whereas a wave V that is not seen until a presentation level of 55 dB suggests a hearing loss approximating 40 dB in the right ear (AD). Reproduced with permission, from Wilson & Nadol Jr. *Quick Reference to Ear, Nose, and Throat Disorders*. Philadelphia: JB Lippincott, 1983

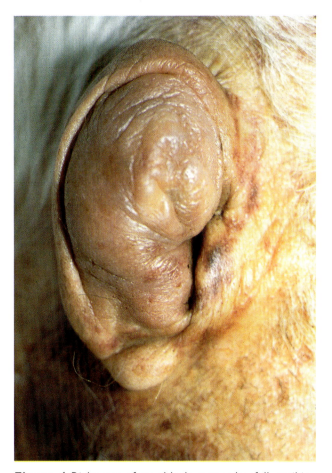

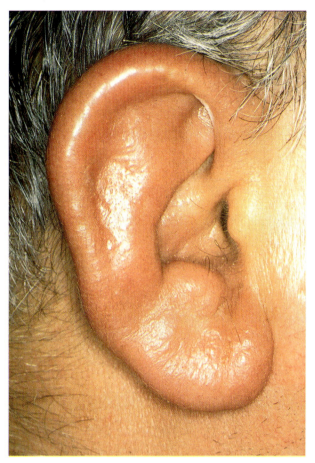

Figure 4 Right ear of an elderly man who fell, striking his head and ear. A hematoma completely occupies the cartilaginous portion of the pinna, indicated by the purplish swelling. The blood in the subperichondrial plane is disrupting the vascular supply of the pinna cartilage from its overlying perichondrium. Hematoma aspiration, using a sterile technique, followed by compression dressing, may be sufficient treatment. On some occasions, repeated aspiration or even more vigorous drainage procedures may be required, along with antibiotic therapy. If left untreated, the underlying cartilage may disintegrate, leaving a 'cauliflower ear'

Figure 5 Cellulitis of the pinna manifests as erythema of the pinna with blunting of the normal topography. Cellulitis may be provoked by trauma or it may arise in association with external otitis. The causative organism is usually either *Staphylococcus aureus* or *Pseudomonas aeruginosa*. Treatment requires intravenous administration of antibiotics and, occasionally, surgical incision and drainage

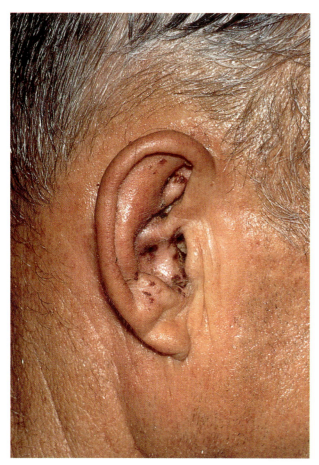

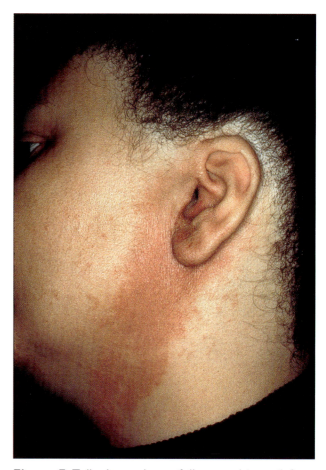

Figure 6 Herpes zoster oticus (Ramsay Hunt syndrome) is a herpesvirus polyneuritis with characteristic pain, and a vesicular outbreak in the external auditory canal and pinna, as seen here. Facial paralysis and evidence of inner ear involvement, with sensorineural hearing loss and vertigo, frequently accompany the vesicular outbreak or follow several days later. Herpesviruses may remain dormant within ganglion cells and cause vesicular disruption when the host is under stress or immunocompromised. Topical therapy usually suffices. High-dose corticosteroid and acyclovir therapy may be helpful in improving the recovery from facial paralysis and hearing loss, although the prognosis is generally poor

Figure 7 Tell-tale erythema follows a drip trail from the auditory canal onto the skin of the neck, suggesting that the patient is allergic to the constituents of an oto-topical antibiotic or wax-removal preparation. A simple test for such hypersensitivity is to place a few drops of the suspect solution onto an adhesive strip, then apply the strip to the skin of the forearm. The finding of erythema 24–48 h later indicates an allergic reaction

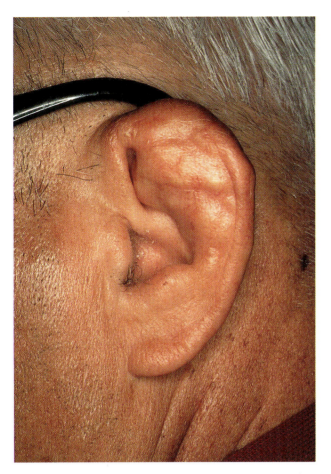

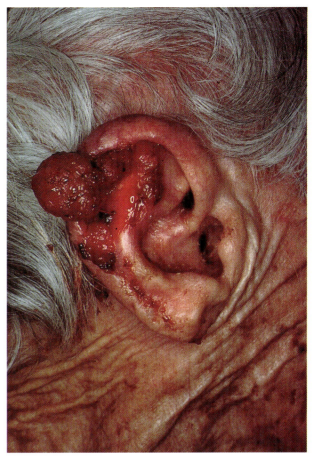

Figure 8 Gouty tophi (deposits of uric acid crystals) in the helix of the pinna. At this site, these well-recognized phenomena of the great toe are generally painless, unlike Winkler's disease, which is characterized by a painful nodule of the pinna. No treatment, other than for the underlying gout, is required

Figure 9 Squamous cell carcinoma (seen here) and basal cell carcinoma are the most common cancers of the pinna and external auditory canal, and are usually associated with a history of chronic sun exposure. Depending on the size and extent of the lesion, simple wedge resection or a complete auriculectomy, neck dissection and radiation therapy may be required for treatment

Figure 10 External otitis, or 'swimmer's ear', is particularly prevalent in the summer, and manifests as an extraordinarily tender and erythematous external auditory canal. Maceration with water (from swimming) or trauma (from cotton-tipped applicators) render the canal prone to infection usually by *S. aureus* or *P. aeruginosa*. After thorough removal of debris from the canal, the typical case responds readily to ototopical antibiotic drops, although narcotic analgesics may be required for a few days to alleviate the discomfort, and no water should be allowed to enter the ear. If there is fever or adenopathy, systemic antibiotics should also be administered. In some cases, the canal may be obliterated by edema, requiring placement of a wick for delivery of antibiotic drops. Intravenous antibiotic therapy is mandatory if there is accompanying cellulitis of the pinna (see Figure 5). Courtesy of E. and K. Yanagisawa; reproduced with permission, from Hughes & Pensak, *Clinical Otology, 2nd edn*. New York: Thieme, 1997

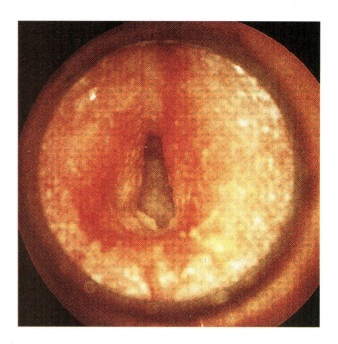

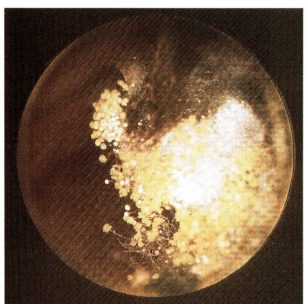

Figure 11 External otitis may be due to fungal infection, most commonly *Aspergillus niger* and *Candida* spp. Canal debris reveals either the fluffy mycelia interspersed with black patches that is typical of *A. niger,* or the thick pasty appearance of *Candida*. Fungal infections may be iatrogenic as a result of extended use of antibacterial ototopical agents. Antifungal drops are indicated. Courtesy of E. and K. Yanagisawa; reproduced with permission, from Hughes & Pensak, *Clinical Otology, 2nd edn*. New York: Thieme, 1997

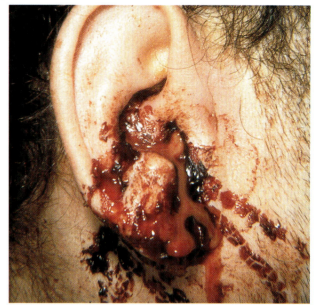

Figure 12 Malignant (or necrotizing) external otitis. This potentially deadly skull-base osteomyelitis occurs in diabetic or immunocompromised subjects and is always due to infection by *P. aeruginosa*. The hallmark clinical finding is granulation tissue at the inferior aspect of the junction of the bony and cartilaginous portions of the external auditory canal. Aggressive long-term therapy with antipseudomonal antibiotics, both systemic and topical, is mandatory, with surgical debridement of devitalized bone as necessary. Poor prognostic signs include facial paralysis and involvement of the lower cranial nerves (IX–XII)

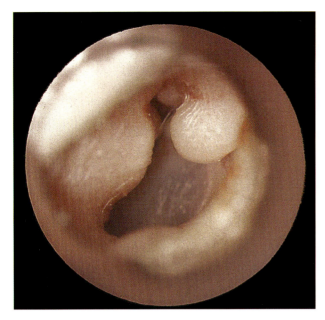

Figure 13 Exostoses or bony excrescences of varying size are seen in the ear canal most commonly in swimmers or surfers (hence, 'surfer's ears'); they are usually bilateral and multiple. It is thought that cold water causes 'refrigeration' periostitis, causing the canal periosteum to lay down a lamella of new bone. Exostoses may grow to such a size as to block the egress of debris from the canal, and lead to recurrent external otitis or conductive hearing loss. Barring such complications, they are to be viewed as a curiosity on physical examination

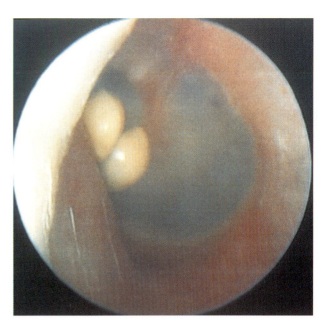

Figure 14 These seeds, placed by a child in the external auditory canal of his left ear, were removed by gentle suction supplemented by microscopic visualization. Insects may also be found in the canal; in such cases, it is easier to 'drown' the insect with mineral oil or ototopical drops before extraction by aspiration

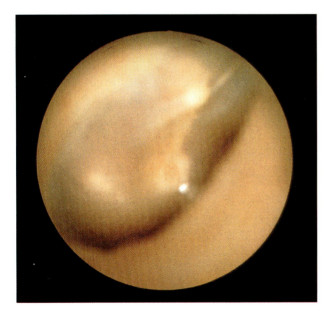

Figure 15 Right ear. The normal tympanic membrane is usually gray and translucent. The lateral process of the malleus forms the prominent knob superiorly and, continuing inferiorly, the stria mallearis (the manubrium seen through the tympanic membrane) ends at the umbo, or distal tip of the manubrium. Superior to the lateral process of the malleus is Schrapnell's membrane, part of the lateral wall of the attic. It is important to visualize the attic region as cholesteatomas may originate at this site and extend silently into the superior recesses of the attic. Anteroinferior to the eardrum is the anterior bulge of the external auditory canal, which varies in prominence from one individual to another. Occasionally, such a bulge may hide a small tympanic membrane perforation. Posteroinferior to the umbo and close to the posterior wall of the external auditory canal, there is often a dark semicircular area, the niche of the round window which houses the round window membrane

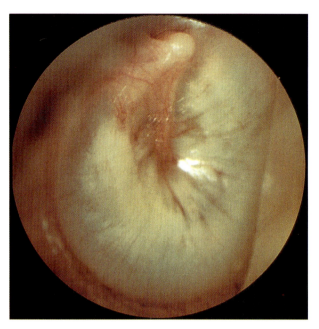

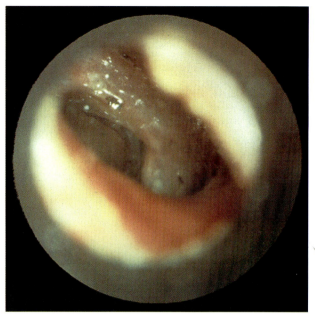

Figure 16 Right ear. In this 'pearly' normal variant, although the usual translucence of the tympanic membrane is diminished, the landmarks are distinguishable and normal

Figure 17 Left ear. Perforation of the tympanic membrane may be caused by trauma, especially from cotton-tipped applicators, or infection. In addition to pain and bleeding from the ear, there may be an associated conductive hearing loss, depending on the size and location of the perforation. If acute, it may be possible to coapt the margins of the perforation to accelerate the healing process. In any case, water precautions and, if the perforation is due to a penetrating foreign body or associated with water entry or infection, ototopical antibiotics are recommended. In most cases, perforations heal spontaneously over the course of a month or so

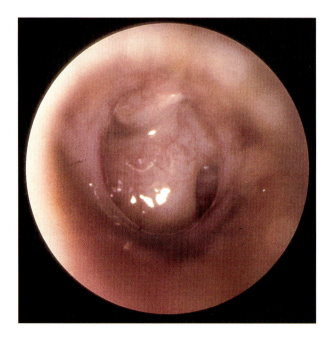

Figure 18 Left ear. Nearly total tympanic membrane perforation. There is little chance of spontaneous healing. The large size of this perforation as well as the exposure of the round window niche predict nearly complete conductive hearing loss

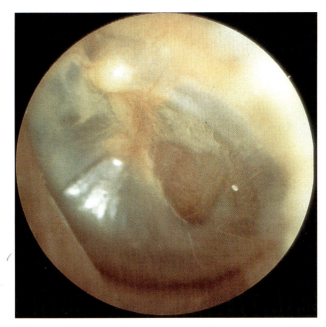

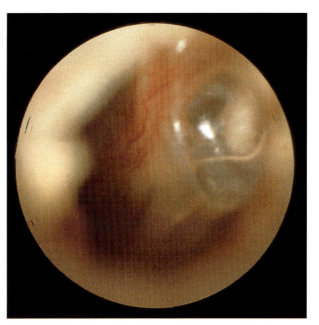

Figure 19 Left ear. In the posteroinferior aspect of this tympanic membrane is a triangular area sealed by a thin replacement membrane, representing a healed perforation. Usually, the tympanic membrane reconstitutes all three layers – outer squamous epithelial, middle fibrous and medial mucosal – in the course of healing a perforation. On occasion, however, the fibrous layer fails to regenerate, leaving a thin 'monomeric' membrane, as seen here

Figure 20 Left ear. In this case, although the tympanic membrane perforation has healed, the replacement membrane is not only thin, but retracted and adherent to the long process of the incus (posterior to the manubrium). It is likely that erosion of the incus, as well as crusting and cholesteatoma formation, will eventually develop in such a situation, leading many otologists to recommend repair with cartilage (cartilage tympanoplasty) even though hearing may be normal or good

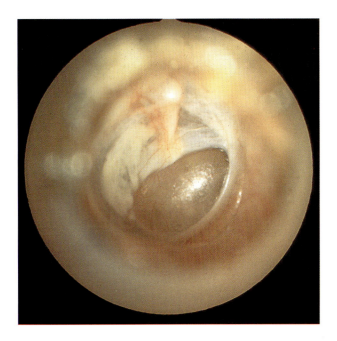

Figure 21 Right ear. In the case shown here, a relatively large anteroinferior perforation has healed, leaving a replacement membrane. The posterior rim of the neomembrane is tympanosclerotic, thickened by fibrous tissue embedded with calcium. Such tympanosclerotic plaques may be large enough to interfere with normal tympanic membrane vibration and mimic a cholesteatoma. However, on pneumatic otoscopy, the tympanosclerotic plaque moves as the tympanic membrane moves, which does not occur with a cholesteatoma

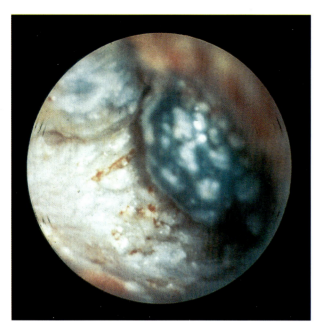

Figure 22 Left ear. Bullous myringitis is an extremely painful infection of the tympanic membrane and external auditory canal thought to be due to either a viral agent or *Mycoplasma pneumoniae*. Lancing the blebs (as seen here) may provide immediate and dramatic relief from pain. Treatment with erythromycin is also recommended

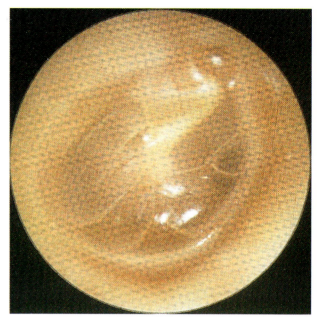

Figure 23 Right ear. Serous otitis refers to a transudate of fluid in the middle ear space due to eustachian tube dysfunction with consequent negative middle ear pressure. This condition is particularly common in infants and children, in whom the eustachian tubes are both narrower in diameter and more horizontally oriented than those of adults and, hence, more prone to obstruction by inflammatory edema or irritation by fluid reflux. Serous otitis may be seen during recovery from acute otitis media or may accompany allergic or infectious rhinosinusitis or nasopharyngitis. In general, serous otitis is bilateral; unilateral serous otitis, especially in an adult, should raise the suspicion of nasopharyngeal tumor. Courtesy of E. and K. Yanagisawa; reproduced with permission, from Hughes & Pensak, *Clinical Otology, 2nd edn.* New York: Thieme, 1997

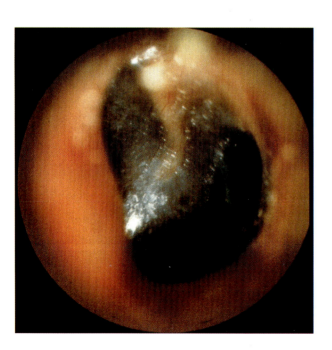

Figure 24 Left ear. On occasion, negative middle ear pressure may be sufficient to disrupt the blood vessels of the middle ear, resulting in a hemorrhagic serous otitis media. This finding may also be seen with closed head trauma, including temporal bone fracture. Immediately after hemorrhage, the blood appears bright red but, as it is metabolized, it darkens, becoming almost black, as seen here

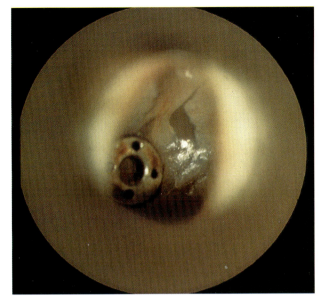

Figure 25 Right ear. Persistent serous otitis media (recurrent acute otitis media) is managed by myringotomy and pressure-equalizing tube insertion (tympanostomy). The Reuter bobbin tube (seen here) usually remains in position for 6–18 months before undergoing spontaneous extrusion. In general, the myringotomy closes as the tube is extruded but, depending on the type of tube used, a permanent perforation may remain

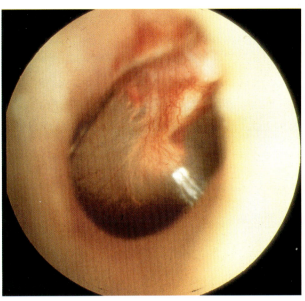

Figure 26 Right ear. Injection surrounding the manubrium and in the posterosuperior quadrant of the drum and canal ('vascular strip' region) indicates early acute otitis media. Antibiotic therapy targets the usual causative organisms, including *Haemophilus influenzae*, *Moraxella catarrhalis* and *Pneumococcus pneumoniae*

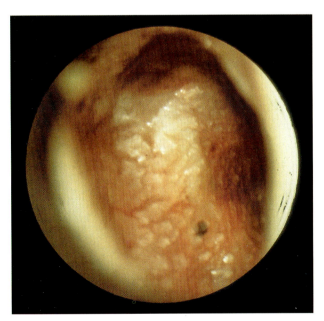

Figure 27 Left ear. A bulging red tympanic membrane is diagnostic of acute otitis media

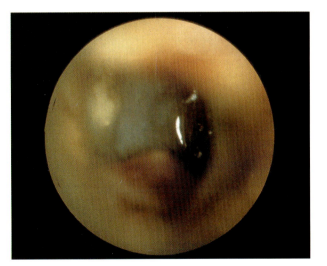

Figure 28 Left ear. No landmarks are distinguishable in this ear, and the polyp in the posterior quadrant raises concern for the presence of cholesteatoma complicating chronic otitis media with tympanic membrane perforation. Initially, the ear is cleaned of debris with the aid of microscopic visualization, and ototopical antibiotics administered. Prior to surgical intervention, audiometric evaluation, perhaps accompanied by temporal bone CT, should be performed

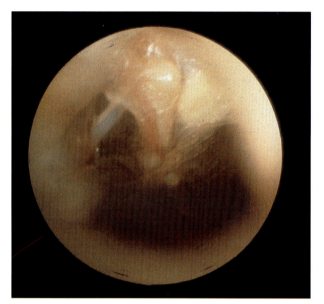

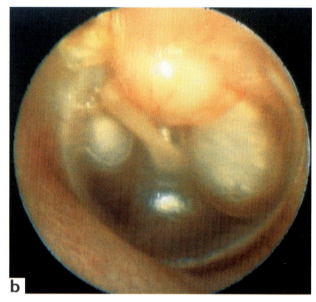

b

Figure 29 Right ear. This small cholesteatoma (ectopic squamous epithelium) is in the anterosuperior quadrant of the middle ear, a site typical of congenital cholesteatomas (arising with no previous history of otitis media), which are thought to develop from embryonic epithelial rests. Surgical excision is required for definitive treatment. The chorda tympani nerve can be seen extending posterior to the manubrium

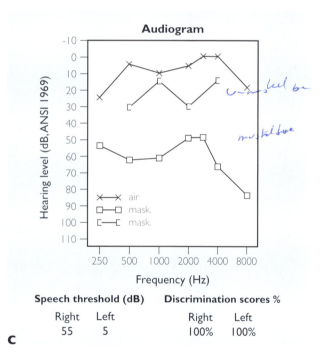

c

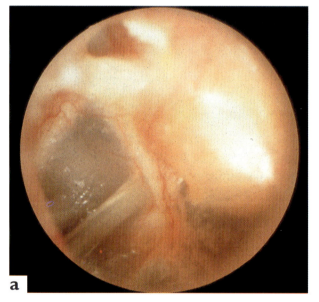

a

Figure 30 Left ear. (a) Attic retraction pocket and perforation resulting in a cholesteatoma that extends into the posterior aspect of the tympanic cavity, classified as a primary acquired cholesteatoma. The degree of extension into the attic and mastoid is determined by imaging studies, preferably temporal bone CT, or by surgical exploration of the attic (atticotomy) and mastoid (mastoidectomy). (b) This large attic cholesteatoma extends inferiorly both anterior and posterior to the manubrium. At surgery, it was noted that the incus and arch of the stapes had been destroyed by the cholesteatoma, which also extended posteriorly into the mastoid. (c) Audiogram showing mixed, predominantly conductive, hearing loss on the right, and normal hearing on the left, the type of hearing loss expected in the ear shown in b

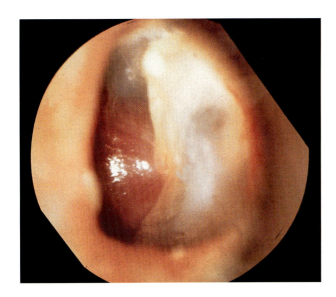

Figure 31 Right ear. The reddish mass in the antero-inferior quadrant of the tympanic cavity is a tympanic paraganglioma (or, more popularly, a glomus tympanicum). Glomus tumors are the most common tumors of the middle ear, and arise from paraganglion cells resting on the promontory of the cochlea in the medial wall of the middle ear and on the dome of the jugular bulb. The tumor here presented with pulsatile tinnitus and a mild conductive hearing loss; surgical excision involved a transcanal tympanotomy. The glomus jugulare, arising from the dome of the jugular bulb, often grows insidiously without causing lower cranial neuropathy until later

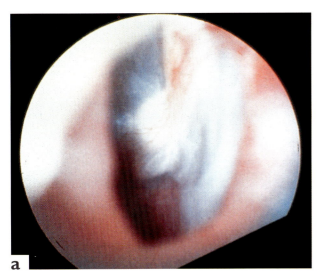

a

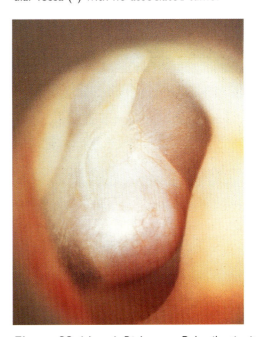

Figure 32 Left ear. (a) A high-riding jugular bulb – one which protrudes from the hypotympanum to rise above the inferior rim of the tympanic membrane – may be mistaken for a glomus tumor. The dark purple color suggests a jugular bulb, but a coronal temporal bone CT (b) establishes the diagnosis by revealing a dehiscent jugular fossa (*) with no associated tumor

b

Figure 33 (above) Right ear. Pulsatile tinnitus may be due to an ectopic internal carotid artery, in this case, running in the anterior portion of the tympanic cavity. NEVER biopsy such a mass! Temporal bone CT delineates the carotid artery canal to determine whether the internal carotid artery is in its normal position

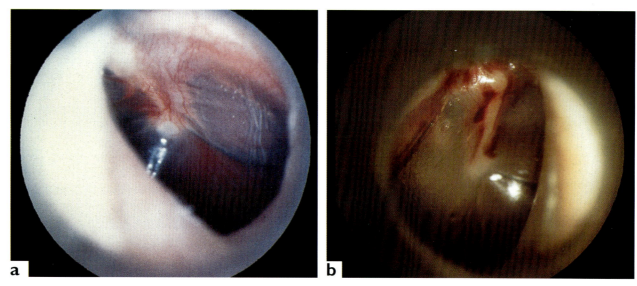

Figure 34 Air travel with a dysfunctional eustachian tube (such as in upper respiratory tract infection) may set the stage for the development of barotitis (or otic barotrauma). The problem arises during descent, when the increasing atmospheric pressure produces a relatively negative middle ear pressure as the eustachian tube is unable to open and equalize pressures. The negative middle ear pressure may become sufficient to tear the blood vessels of the eardrum (a; left ear) and middle ear, resulting in hemotympanum. The patient presents with a blocked ear and a variable degree of hearing loss. Air travel should be avoided until eustachian tube function is recovered. Oral antibiotics are advisable in the face of frank hemotympanum (a) in which an air–blood level is clearly evident. In this right ear (b), there is hemorrhagic streaking of the tympanic membrane with serous effusion due to barotrauma

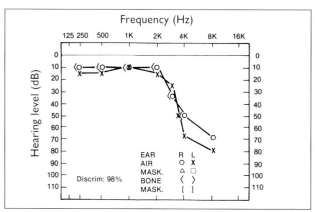

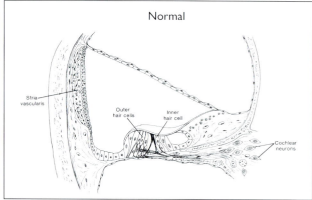

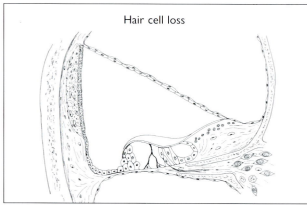

Figure 35 Pattern of hearing loss in sensory presbycusis (upper left) is typified by a sharp drop-off in the high tones with relatively good speech discrimination (98%), a reflection of hair cell loss (lower left) in the base of the cochlea; normal anatomy of the inner ear (upper right). Modified with permission, from *ASHA Reports*, Number 19, 1990

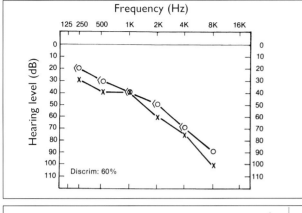

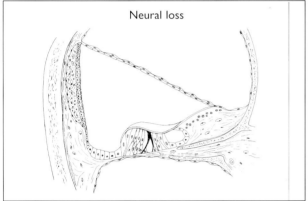

Figure 36 In neural presbycusis, not only is there loss of pure-tone perception, but speech discrimination is also deteriorated (upper), a result of dysfunction (or loss) of hair cells and neural elements in the cochlea (lower). Modified with permission, from *ASHA Reports*, Number 19, 1990

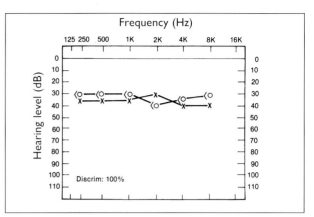

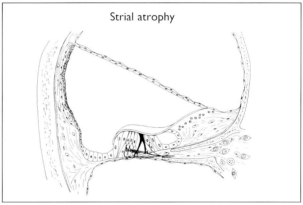

Figure 37 In presbycusis with strial atrophy, there is a relatively flat threshold pattern, and speech discrimination remains excellent until the hearing levels approach approximately 50 dB (upper). This type of presbycusis is thought to stem from dysfunction of the stria vascularis (lower), the 'energy pump' of the cochlea. Modified with permission, from *ASHA Reports*, Number 19, 1990

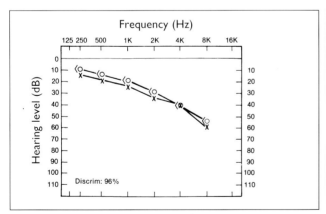

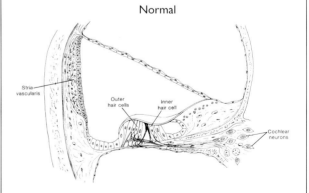

Figure 38 In cochlear conductive presbycusis, thresholds decline progressively throughout the frequency range (left), and speech discrimination (96% in this case) is inversely proportional to the slope of decline. This type of presbycusis is thought to be related to changes in the basilar membrane upon which the hair cells rest (right). Modified with permission, from *ASHA Reports*, Number 19, 1990

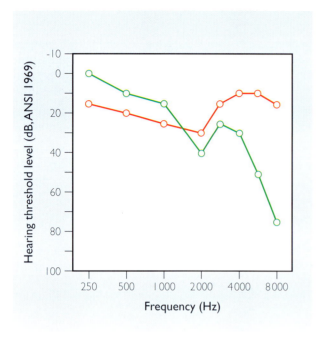

Figure 39 Ototoxic agents initially and most severely affect high-frequency hearing. Systemic ototoxic agents, such as aminoglycosides, cause a relatively symmetrical high-frequency hearing loss. In this case, local application of an aminoglycoside-containing solution in the presence of tympanic membrane perforation was associated with development of a unilateral high-frequency sensorineural hearing loss. Curves 1 (red) and 2 (green) were obtained before and after drop application, respectively

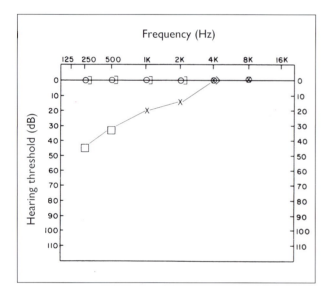

Figure 40 Meniere's disease typically presents with a fluctuating low-frequency sensorineural hearing loss, and may be mimicked by otitis due to syphilis

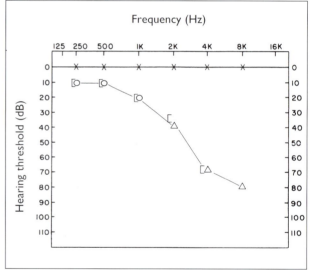

Figure 41 The vast majority of disorders precipitating sensorineural hearing loss affects both ears symmetrically; a notable exception is endolymphatic hydrops (as in Meniere's disease). Detection of an asymmetrical sensorineural hearing loss, especially if associated with poor speech discrimination, should raise suspicion of an acoustic neuroma, a benign tumor arising from the Schwann cells of the vestibular nerve. The tumor may originate either in the cerebellopontine angle (CPA) or in the internal auditory canal with extension into the CPA

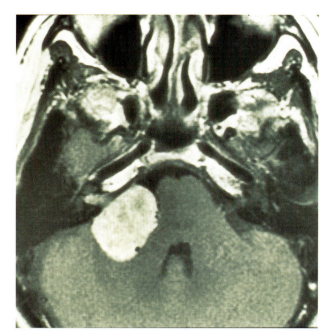

Figure 42 At present, gadolinium-enhanced MRI is the most definitive means for diagnosis of acoustic neuroma

NOSE

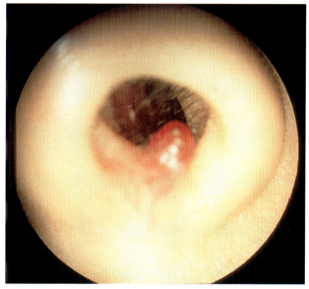

Figure 43 In addition to furuncles (staphylococcal infection of the hair follicles), a variety of true neoplasms, both benign and malignant, may occur in the nasal vestibule. In the case shown here, there is a benign hemangioma in the lateral inferior aspect of the left vestibule. Simple excision is adequate therapy

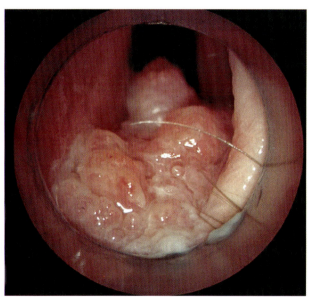

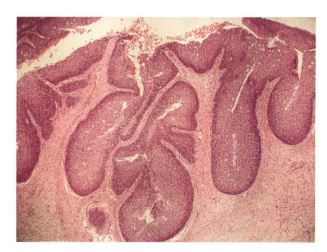

Figure 44 The inverting papilloma, in this case in the nasal vestibule (left), is a benign tumor but, unless completely resected, has a strong propensity for recurrence with local extension and bony destruction that may involve the orbit and anterior cranial fossa. Radiation therapy has been suggested to precipitate malignant degeneration. The low-power histological view (right) shows the characteristic papillomas (H & E stain)

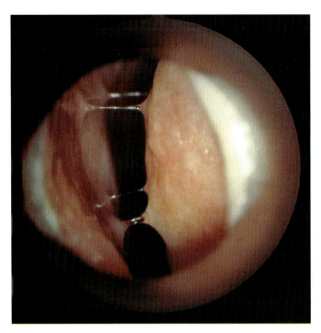

Figure 45 Although crystalline mucus strands, suggesting allergic rhinitis, are seen crossing the nasal cavity, the inferior turbinate (on the right) is of normal size and the nasal airway is patent

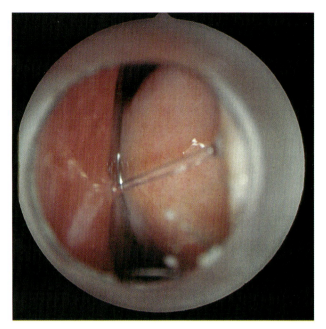

Figure 46 In acute allergic reactions or chronic allergic rhinitis, the turbinates swell to such an extent as to occlude the nasal passages (as seen here). Rhinitis medicamentosa, due to overuse of topical vasoconstrictors such as neosynephrine or oxymetazoline, may also result in turbinate edema. In rhinitis medicamentosa, the vasoconstrictive agents overwhelm normal adrenergic control of the vascular beds of the nasal cavity, disrupt the normal circadian rhythm of swelling and shrinking of the turbinates, and cause nasal obstruction responsive only temporarily to topical vasoconstrictors. Treatment involves discontinuation of topical vasoconstrictors, and substitution of corticosteroid nasal sprays and systemic decongestants. Surgery involving partial resection of the lower one-third of the inferior turbinate is effective in recalcitrant cases (see Figure 48)

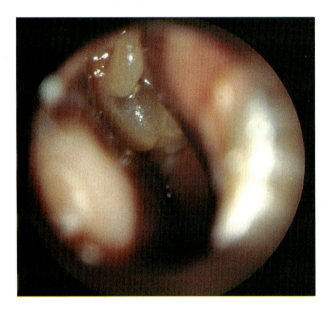

Figure 47 Nasal polyps (above and right) may complicate chronic allergic rhinitis and cause nasal obstruction. The polyps are superior to the inferior turbinate and inferior to the middle turbinate, suggesting egress at the ethmoid sinus. If topical steroids do not eliminate the polyps, then surgical resection (polypectomy or ethmoidectomy) may be required. It is important to determine, using appropriate imaging, that a single 'polyp' is not, in fact, herniated brain substance (encephalocele)

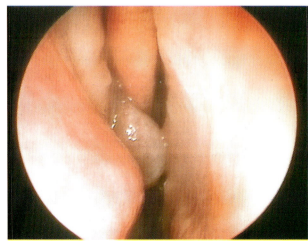

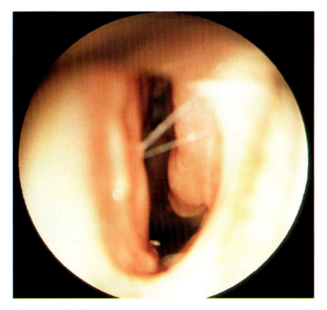

Figure 48 Chronic nasal obstruction due to medically unresponsive turbinate hypertrophy is successfully managed by surgical resection of a portion of the turbinate, the so-called turbinate trim. The example seen here shows good turbinate reduction several weeks after surgery. Turbinate trimming, if overdone, may result in a dry crusty nose

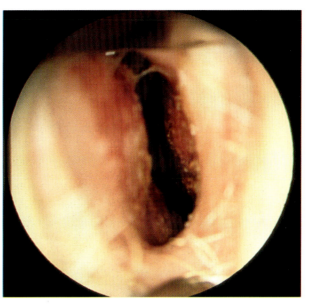

Figure 49 Atrophic rhinitis tends to predominate in postmenopausal women and is idiopathic in most cases. Atrophy of the nasal mucosa leads to a diminished amount of mucus, which dries to form malodorous crusts. Although there is no specific therapy, saline irrigation of the nose may prove helpful

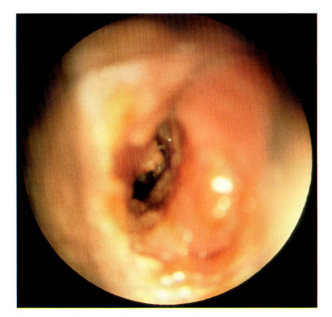

Figure 50 Sarcoidosis is typified by non-caseating granulomas (seen on histopathological examination of biopsy specimens) that may involve the nose. Treatment consists of corticosteroid therapy

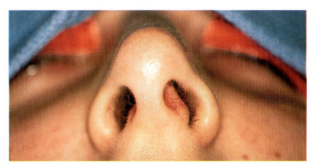

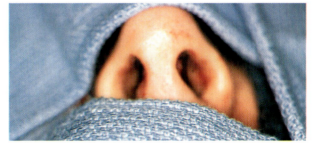

Figure 51 One of the most common abnormalities of the nose is deviation of the nasal septum, usually to the right, although deviation to the left may also occur (upper). If the deviation is sufficient to cause nasal obstruction, septoplasty, or removal of the obstructing portion of the nasal septum (lower), may be curative

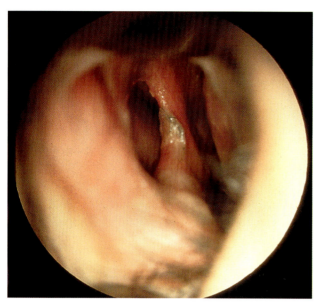
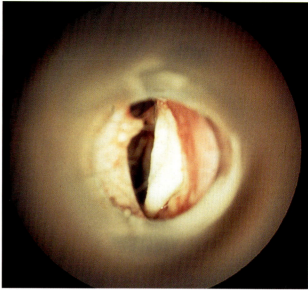

Figure 52 Care must be taken not to separate the septum completely from its perichondrium as the ensuing disruption of blood supply may lead to septal atrophy and an externally evident 'saddle' deformity of the nasal dorsum or perforation of the nasal septum. The latter, which may also be due to cocaine abuse (snorting), causes a site of bleeding and crusting in the nasal septum (left); a septal button seals the perforation (right)

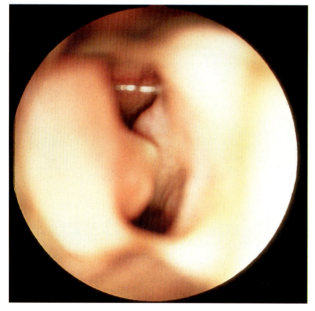

Figure 53 Sluder's headaches, typified by deep pain in the orbit and face, are thought to be related to a high posterior nasal septal spur impinging on the lateral nasal wall. Relief of pain with topical anesthesia of the spur helps to make the diagnosis; surgical resection of the offending spur is effective in alleviating the headache

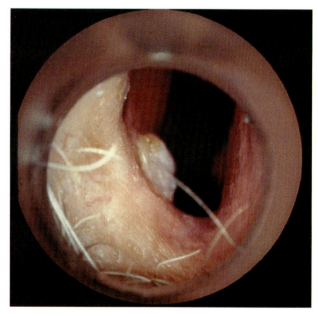

Figure 54 This small sessile papilloma arises from the septum and protrudes into the left nasal cavity. Simple resection is indicated

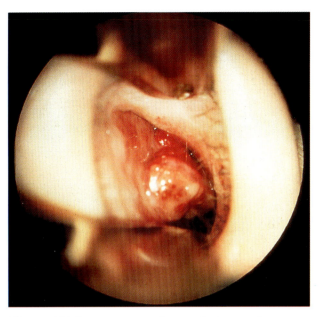

Figure 55 Pyogenic granuloma of the nasal septum. Bacterial invasion facilitated by trauma or irritation of mucous membranes results in a rapidly growing, friable mass. Complete excision is recommended

PARANASAL SINUSES

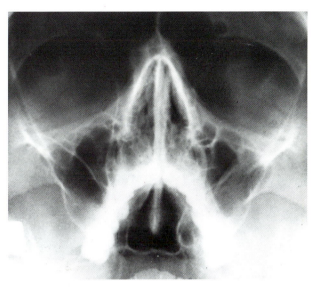

Figure 56 Plane X-ray (normal Water's view) demonstrates the maxillary sinus (above the maxillary teeth) particularly well. Using the 'open-mouth' technique, the sphenoid sinus (below the teeth) is also evaluable

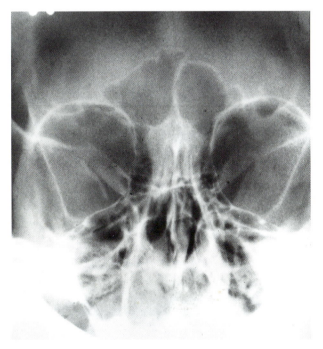

Figure 57 Plane X-ray (Caldwell view) allows evaluation of both the frontal sinuses (above and medial to the orbits) and ethmoid sinuses (between the orbits)

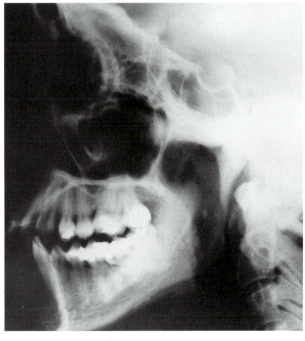

Figure 58 Plane X-ray (lateral view) is useful in the assessment of the frontal, maxillary and sphenoid sinuses as well as the nasopharynx

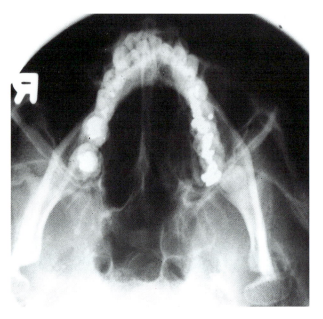

Figure 59 Plane X-ray (base view) enables visualization of the sphenoid and maxillary sinuses. This is useful in the management of acute facial trauma, particularly if there is suspected fracture of the malar eminence

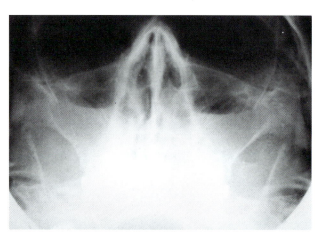

Figure 60 Plane X-ray (Water's view) showing bilateral maxillary sinus air–fluid levels in acute sinusitis. The most common causative organisms include *Streptococcus pneumoniae*, *H. influenzae* and *M. catarrhalis*. Management includes nasal and systemic decongestants, and oral antibiotics

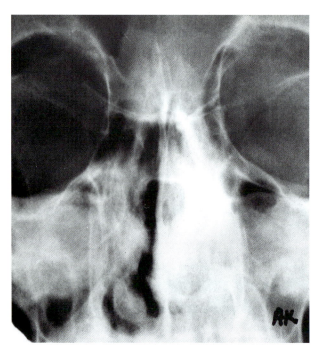

Figure 61 Plane X-ray (Water's view) showing inflammatory polypoid disease that is worse on the left than on the right and, in this case, associated with allergic rhinosinusitis

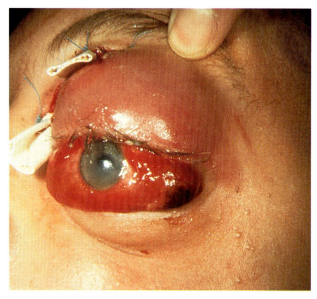

Figure 62 Acute ethmoiditis causes lid edema and erythema which, if left untreated, progresses to severe orbital celllulitis (seen here). Emergency surgical drainage by ethmoidectomy (two Penrose drains are visible at the medial/superior aspect of the eye) together with intensive intravenous antibiotic delivery comprise the appropriate therapy

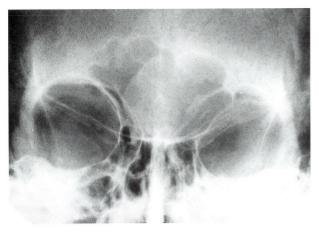

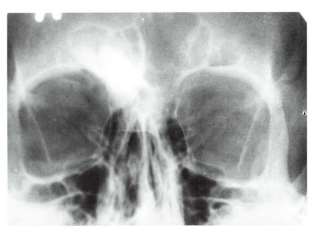

Figure 63 Plane X-ray (Caldwell view) showing opacification of the left frontal sinus due to a mucocele, an expanding mucosal cyst filled with mucus. As seen here, a mucocele may erode the bony margins of the sinus and encroach upon the adjacent orbit. An infected mucocele is called a pyocele. Management of a mucopyocele involves surgical resection of the diseased sinus tissue by endoscopy, with osteoplastic frontal sinus obliteration in recalcitrant cases

Figure 64 Plane X-ray (Caldwell view) showing intense opacification in the right frontal sinus due to an osteoma. With expansion, this benign bony tumor may lead to displacement of the globe or even proptosis. Surgical excision by osteoplastic frontal sinus obliteration is curative

ORAL CAVITY AND PHARYNX

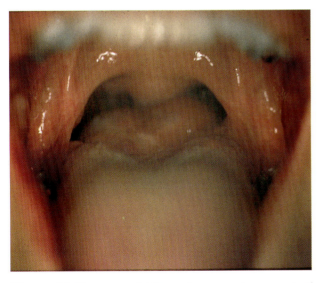

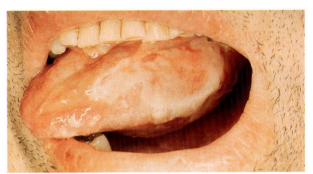

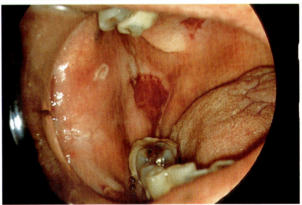

Figure 65 The mass visible at the posterior aspect of the tongue, near the region of the circumvallate papillae, is thyroid tissue that has failed to complete its embryological descent into the neck. This tissue may represent the patient's only thyroid tissue

Figure 66 These bullae of pemphigus vulgaris on the lateral tongue (upper) are painless, but rupture to leave painful ulcers. These bullae are formed intraepidermally whereas, in pemphigoid, the apparently similar bullae are formed subepidermally. Formerly a lethal condition, pemphigus is now managed by systemic corticosteriods and topical treatment of the oral lesions. Pemphigus vulgaris on the right posterior buccal mucosa (lower)

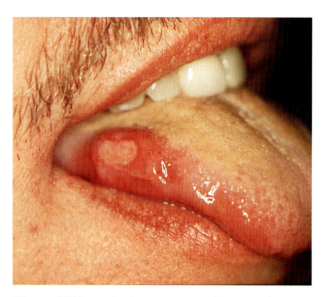

Figure 67 Herpetic glossitis is part of an acute herpetic stomatitis. The vesicles rupture within around 24 h to leave behind shallow yellowish ulcers which heal over approximately 1 week. On occasions, the lesions may be painful; symptomatic therapy is then indicated. This self-limiting disease usually runs its course over a period of 3 weeks

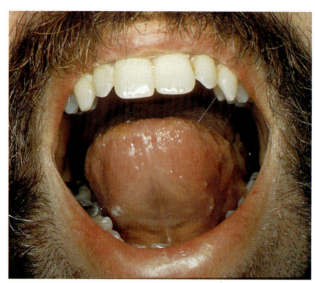

Figure 68 Acute edema of the tongue may be related to allergy, angioneurotic edema or, more recently, angiotensin-converting enzyme (ACE) inhibitor therapy. Management in mild cases, as seen here, consists of corticosteroids and antihistamines. In more severe cases, intubation by tracheotomy may be necessary to manage airways obstruction

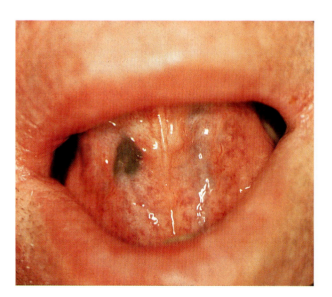

Figure 69 Although worrisome in appearance, this amalgam tattoo represents a harmless souvenir of dental work

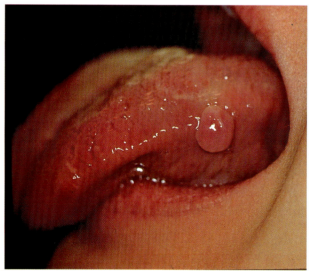

Figure 70 This mass on the lateral aspect of the tongue is a fibroma; simple excision suffices as therapy

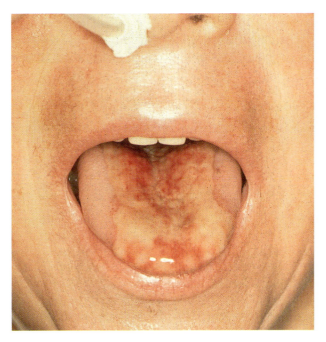

Figure 71 Caustic burns of the tongue generally stem from alkali ingestion. Concomitant esophageal burns, which constitute a more difficult management problem, must be suspected in such a scenario (note the nasogastric tube *in situ*)

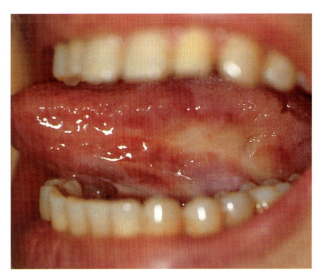

Figure 72 The vast majority of lingual cancers are squamous cell carcinomas, and the lateral aspect of the middle third of the tongue is the most common location. Due to the bilateral lymphatic drainage of this part of the tongue, management requires radical surgery. In this case, barring other involvement of the aerodigestive tract, hemiglossectomy with neck dissection and subsequent radiation therapy to both sides of the neck are recommended

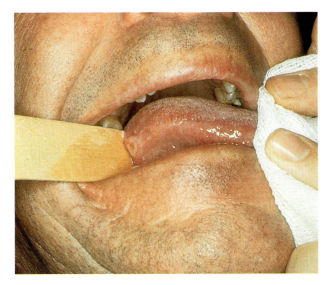

Figure 73 In contrast to the ectodermal derivation of the anterior tongue, the posterior tongue is derived from endoderm. This differing embryological origin may account for the more invasive anaplastic and metastatic characteristics of posterior tongue carcinomas. Surgery and / or radiation therapy are treatment options

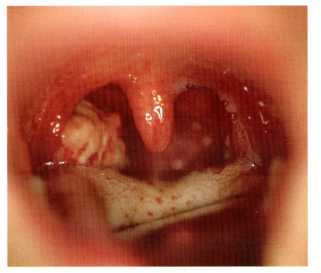

Figure 74 Acute exudative (palatine) tonsillitis may be associated with a generalized (β-hemolytic) streptococcal pharyngitis; alternative etiological organisms include staphylococci and *H. influenzae*. Penicillin therapy has been considered curative, but emerging resistance even among streptococcal strains suggests the need to reassess initial therapy on the basis of clinical, as well as culture and sensitivity, results

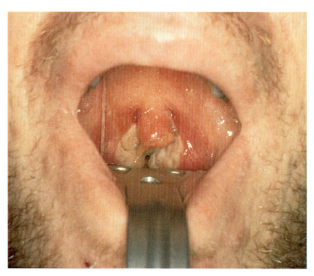

Figure 75 Acute viral tonsillitis responds to symptomatic therapy. The usefulness of antibiotic therapy in preventing secondary bacterial infection has not been determined

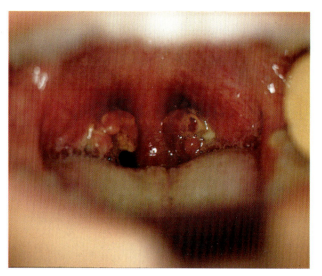

Figure 76 Infectious mononucleosis may produce an impressive tonsillitis. A complete blood count with differential demonstrates atypical lymphocytes before the heterophil antigen test becomes positive. Hepatic and splenic involvement must be assessed. Therapy consists of corticosteriods for edema and antibiotics for secondary bacterial infection. Ampicillin should be avoided as it precipitates a skin rash in this clinical setting

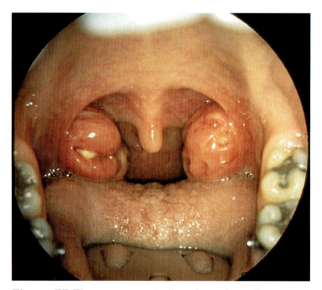

Figure 77 These symmetrically enlarged tonsils are typical of chronic cryptic tonsillitis. β-Lactamase-producing organisms in the depths of the crypts may contribute to the antibiotic resistance of infecting organisms, thereby complicating therapy. Tonsillectomy is curative

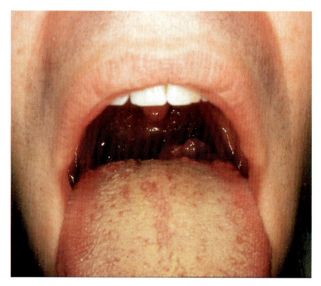

Figure 78 The erythematous mass at the left posterior tongue represents an acutely inflamed lingual tonsil. Etiological organisms and treatment are the same as for palatine tonsillitis (see Figure 74)

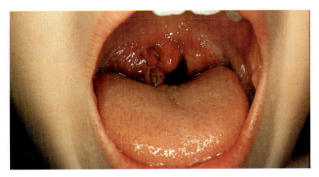

Figure 79 Although acute tonsillitis may be asymmetrical, such a finding should also raise suspicion of an underlying malignancy. This patient has, in addition to bilateral chronic tonsillitis, an underlying lymphoma (on the patient's right)

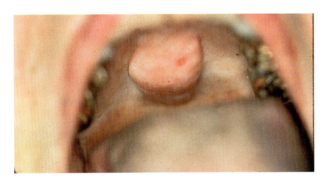

Figure 81 A torus palatinus is a midline osteoma. A similar growth may arise on the lingual surface of the mandible, which is then referred to as a torus mandibularis. Little difficulty is caused by such lesions unless the patient is a denture candidate

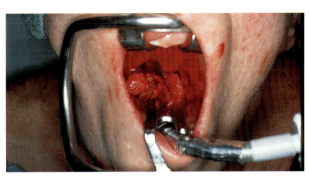

Figure 80 Well over 90% of all tonsillar cancers are of squamous cell origin, as is this large right-sided tumor. The typical patient, including those with head and neck squamous cell carcinomas, usually has a long-term history of smoking and alcohol consumption, and complains of a chronic sore throat that may radiate as far as the ear. For small lesions, radiation therapy may suffice but, with larger lesions, wide-field resection including the surrounding soft tissue, mandible and draining lymph nodes followed by flap reconstruction is necessary

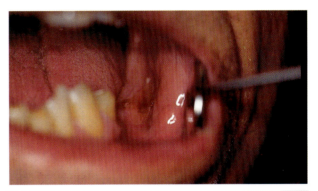

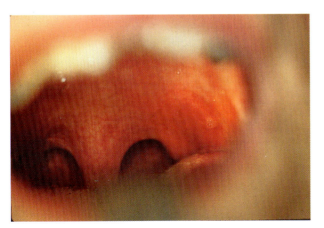

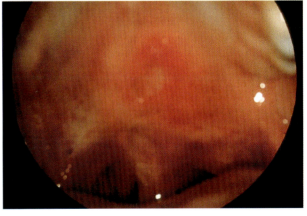

Figure 82 Ruptured bulla of pemphigoid on the left soft palate (left). Pemphigoid differs from pemphigus vulgaris by having a benign course and, on histopathological examination, subepidermal bullae. Treatment is with corticosteroids. Pemphigoid of the right cheek (upper right) and aphthous stomatitis (canker sore) of the soft palate (lower right) are ulcerating lesions with a 2–4-day course of pain followed by a healing period lasting several days. Symptomatic therapy, such as anesthetic lozenges or topical steroids in Orabase®, is recommended

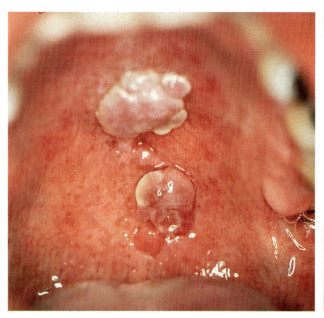
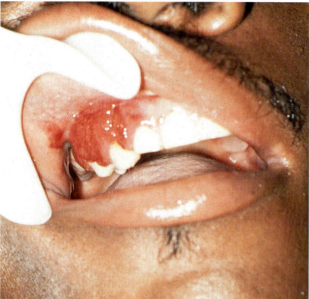

Figure 83 A variety of oral lesions may be seen in the HIV-infected population. This patient with AIDS (left) has lesions of Kaposi's sarcoma on the roof of the mouth whereas, in another AIDS patient (right), Kaposi's sarcoma involves the gingival mucosa

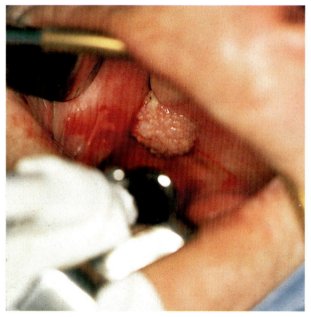
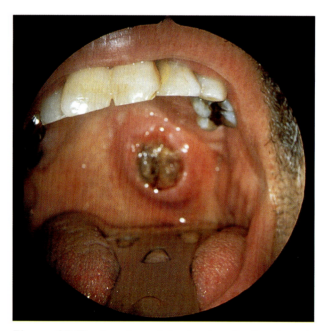

Figure 84 Intraoperative view of an exophytic squamous cell carcinoma of the right hard palate. Wide resection with prosthetic reconstruction is the recommended treatment

Figure 85 The junction of the hard and soft palates is characterized by an abundance of minor salivary glands. In this patient, a large adenoid cystic carcinoma is arising from this junctional area. Radical resection is required for management of such lesions, but the prognosis is poor because of the neural invasion and spread typical of this type of cancer

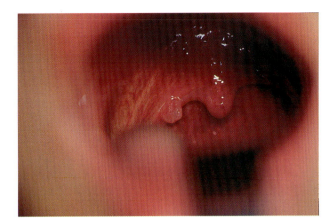

Figure 86 This wart-like growth on the right soft palate is a papilloma. Therapy consists of complete local excision

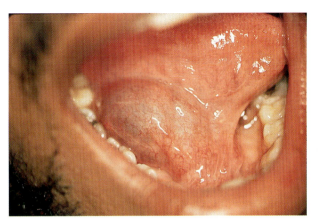

Figure 87 A ranula (L, 'little frog') is a mucus-filled cyst resulting from the breakdown of the sublingual gland. Complete excision, a technically challenging procedure because of the thin wall of the cyst, is recommended

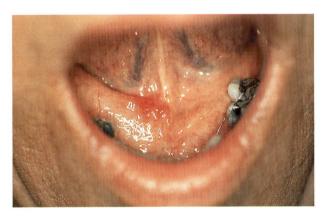

Figure 88 The reddish area on the right at the base of the frenulum near the opening of the submandibular gland duct is a small squamous cell carcinoma. Wide local resection is recommended for such a lesion

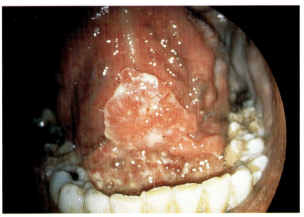

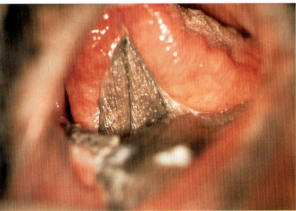

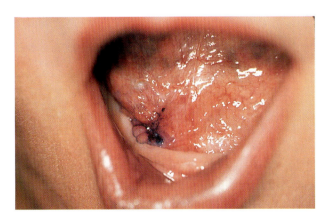

Figure 89 This slightly larger squamous cell carcinoma has a similar location to the lesion in Figure 88. Toluidine blue staining helps to delineate the full extent of the tumor prior to resection

Figure 90 This large squamous cell carcinoma of the floor of the mouth (upper) was treated by floor-of-mouth resection, in-continuity upper-neck dissection and marginal mandibulectomy. Flaps may be used to reconstruct the defect; in this case (lower), a pectoralis major myocutaneous flap has been used

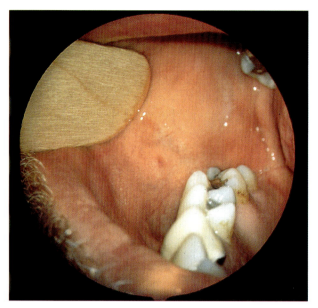

Figure 91 Erythema of the punctum of the parotid duct is typically present in mumps parotitis

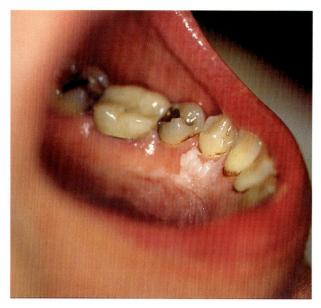

Figure 92 This white patch (leukoplakia) on the gingival mucosa is a premalignant lesion commonly encountered in smokers. Surgical excision is recommended

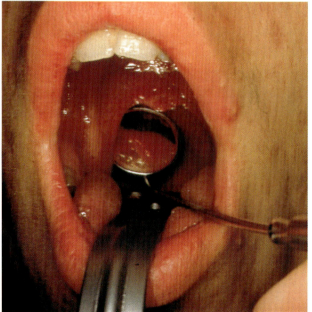

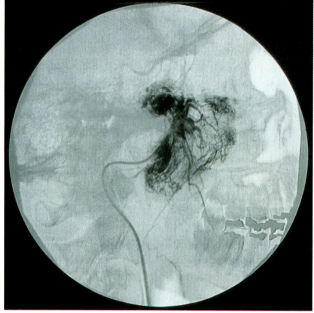

Figure 93 The nasopharyngeal tumor seen in this mirror examination is a juvenile angiofibroma (left). These tumors are highly vascular and typically occur in adolescent males. Presenting symptoms are nasal obstruction and epistaxis. Angiography delineates the extent of the tumor, and preoperative embolization of the tumor blood supply facilitates the recommended surgical resection. The intense blush evident on the arteriogram (right; lateral view) was seen following selective injection of the internal maxillary artery and delineates the extent of the juvenile angiofibroma

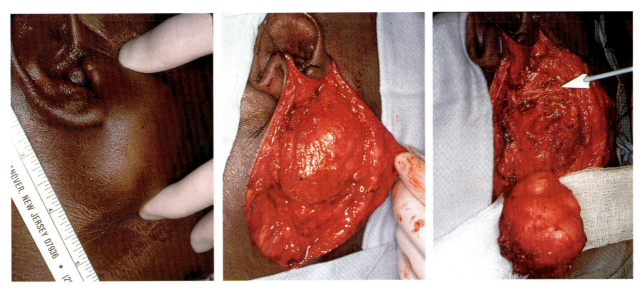

Figure 94 The parotid gland is the most common site of salivary gland tumors, and the vast majority of parotid gland tumors are benign mixed tumors. These slow-growing, painless tumors may become sizable (left). Wide excision that includes a cuff of normal parotid tissue (middle) should prevent tumor seeding and recurrence. The tumor is excised (right) after ensuring that the facial nerve has been preserved (arrowed)

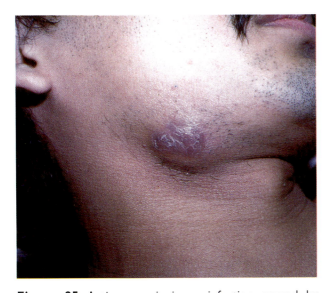

Figure 95 Actinomycosis is an infection caused by *Actinomyces israelii* which develops at or near the mandible after dental work or other trauma. An abscess is formed and followed by draining sinuses. The finding of 'sulfur granules' on biopsy (or positive cultures) is diagnostic. High-dose penicillin is recommended

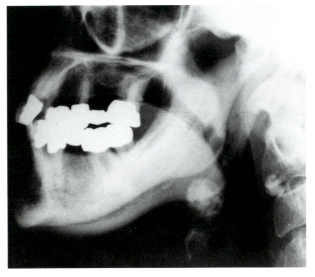

Figure 96 The vast majority of salivary duct stones (sialoliths) arise in the submandibular gland, and cause swelling and pain during eating. Diagnosis is facilitated when the stone is radiopaque, as seen in this X-ray. Treatment depends on the size and location of the stone, and ranges from simple 'milking' of the stone from the duct to submandibular gland excision

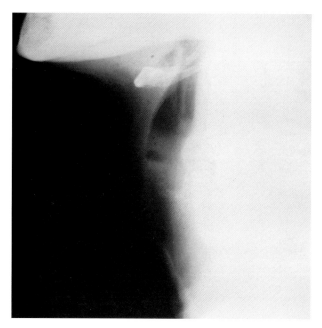

Figure 97 X-ray (lateral view) of a normal neck

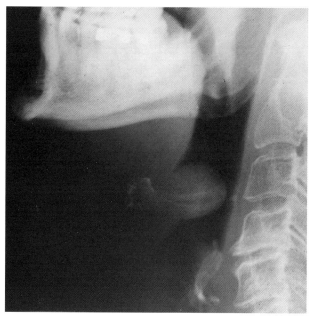

Figure 98 X-ray (lateral view) of acute epiglottitis, a disease usually of young children, but also seen in adults. The 'thumbprint' sign reflects swelling of the epiglottis (arrowed), and its impact on the airways is evident. The widespread use of the *H. influenzae* vaccine has contributed to the decline in the incidence of this disorder

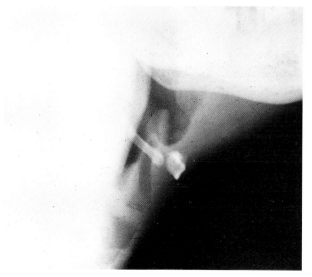

Figure 99 X-ray of a retropharyngeal abscess, defined radiographically by loss of the normal lordotic curve of the cervical spine (straightening of the neck). The thickness of the retropharyngeal tissue, normally no more than one-third of the anteroposterior diameter of the cervical body, is also increased. In young children, pharyngeal infection with suppurative adenopathy is causative whereas, in adults, penetrating visceral injury is the usual cause. Airways distress and dysphagia should prompt medical attention. Incision and drainage of the abscess with broad-spectrum antibiotics comprise the recommended therapy

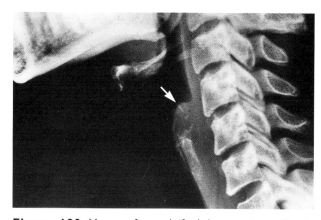

Figure 100 X-ray of a calcified larynx, immediately above which lies a fish bone, presenting as a hyperdense sliver (arrowed), impaled in the mucosa over the arytenoid process of the larynx. Due to their low calcium content, fish bones are usually not well visualized whereas chicken bones, with their higher calcium content, are more readily seen. Operative direct laryngoscopy under general anesthesia is required for extraction. If neglected, this bone could precipitate retropharyngeal abscess formation

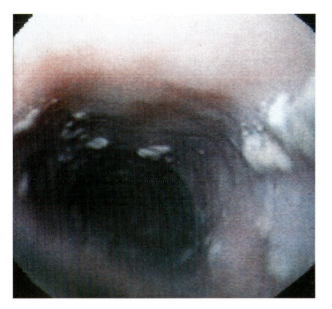

Figure 101 Fiberoptic esophagoscopy of esophagitis due to *Candida albicans* accompanied by severe dysphagia. Such a finding should raise suspicion of HIV infection, as was the case in this patient, and is managed with oral and systemic antifungal agents

LARYNX

In all of the following rigid endoscopic photographs, the top of the image corresponds to the posterior aspect of the larynx, and the right side of the larynx is to the left

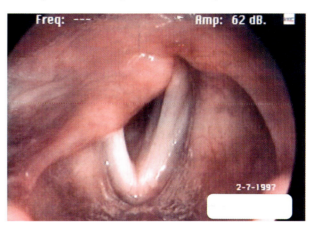

Figure 102 Unilateral vocal cord paralysis with the paralyzed right vocal fold lying laterally. A common presenting complaint is a hoarse breathy voice following an upper respiratory tract infection. Any patient with protracted hoarseness (>6–8 weeks) should undergo further evaluation, including imaging of the course of the vagus and recurrent laryngeal nerves by either CT or MRI. The differential diagnosis of vocal cord paralysis includes head and neck carcinoma, skull-base tumors, thyroid carcinoma, cervical, mediastinal or surgical (post-thyroidectomy) trauma and diabetic neuropathy. In most cases, no cause is found even after careful evaluation and the paralysis is then classified as 'idiopathic'. Current management options include medialization of the vocal cord by thyroplasty or arytenoid adduction, resulting in a voice of good quality maintained in the long term

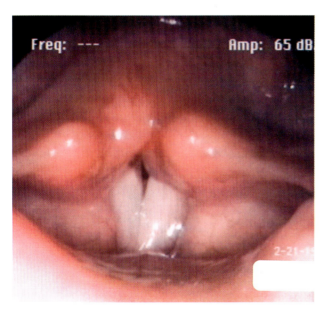

Figure 103 Bilateral vocal cord paralysis following bilateral recurrent laryngeal nerve injury during total thyroidectomy. Both vocal cords are in a midline position, causing airways obstruction. Vocal quality remains good due to the proximity of the static vocal cords, which allows them to vibrate in response to the air stream. Tracheotomy may be required in such cases to provide an adequate airway. Surgical trauma, such as thyroidectomy or posterior cranial fossa/skull base surgery, is the most common cause of bilateral vocal cord paralysis. Proper evaluation includes CT or MRI of the course of the vagus and recurrent laryngeal nerves, with special attention to the brain stem and thyroid gland. Definitive management entails CO_2 laser arytenoidectomy or cordotomy which, however, results in deterioration of the voice

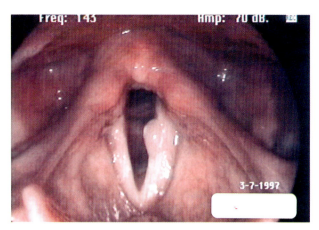

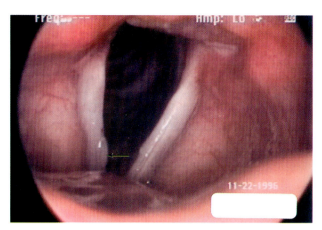

Figure 104 Isolated laryngeal papilloma of the left vocal fold. These usually cause chronic hoarseness of gradual onset, affect both adults and children, and are associated with type-specific human papillomaviruses. Current management involves microlaryngeal removal with a cold knife and CO_2 laser. Laryngeal papillomata tend to recur probably because of their viral etiology. With excision, there is usually an improvement in voice quality, which worsens with recurrence. It is not unusual for patients to undergo multiple excisions prior to cure. On rare occasions, there may be spontaneous resolution

Figure 105 Vocal fold cysts are usually isolated lesions occurring at any location on the vocal cord (in this case, on the anterior aspect of the right vocal fold), and are frequently associated with vocal abuse and possibly gastroesophageal reflux. As with other mass lesions of the vocal folds, they cause chronic hoarseness. Evaluation is limited to a thorough history of vocal use and examination with videostroboscopy. Management includes voice therapy with special attention to vocal hygiene. Surgical excision is usually necessary

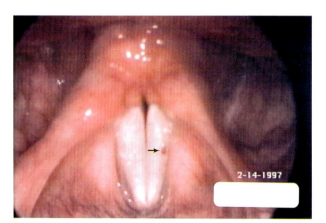

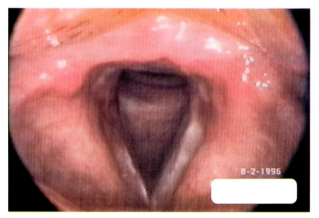

Figure 106 Isolated cysts of the vocal fold are most often associated with feeding blood vessels which rupture readily with trauma, such as voicing or coughing, resulting in a hemorrhage within the cyst (arrowed). Hemorrhagic cysts are diagnosed by videostroboscopy, and managed initially by observation and voice rest. The hemorrhagic component generally resolves, but the cyst persists. Such cysts are best managed by excision, using suspension microlaryngoscopy and coagulation of the feeding vessel(s) by a CO_2 laser. An excellent voice is anticipated after cyst excision

Figure 107 Hemorrhage of the vocal fold is rare. The patient typically suddenly becomes hoarse after shouting, singing with a cold, deceleration injury or aggressive sneezing. Laryngeal examination is diagnostic. Usually, only one vocal fold is involved (in this case, the right fold). It is thought that an aggressive adduction force in the setting of dilated blood vessels results in hemorrhage into the superficial lamina propria. As a rule, the hemorrhage resolves spontaneously. Voice rest is recommended in the acute phase, and outcomes are typically excellent, although a professional singer may notice a substantial long-term deterioration in range and endurance

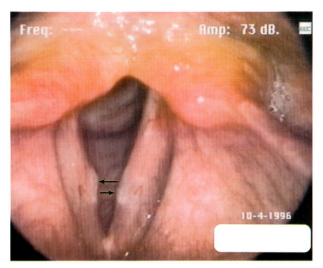

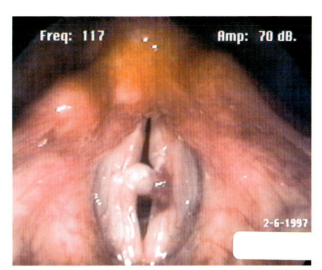

Figure 108 Classically, vocal nodules (arrowed) are bilateral lesions involving the vibratory surface of the vocal folds at the junction of the anterior one-third and posterior two-thirds. These lesions interfere with vocal fold vibration, causing hoarseness. Nodules are seen in patients who misuse their voices, such as cheerleaders and drill sergeants. The appearance of nodules is diagnostic, although they may be mistaken for bilateral cysts. Vocal nodules are best managed by voice therapy with attention to improved voice-use habits. Shouting or talking in a noisy environment without amplification as well as smoking should be strictly avoided. With good voice therapy, approximately 80% of patients resolve their nodules. If voice therapy fails, vocal nodules can be excised by a direct microlaryngoscopic approach. Voice outcomes after surgical excision are variable, but usually excellent

Figure 109 Vocal fold polyps are usually single, broad- or narrow-based, soft, gray lesions occurring almost anywhere on the vocal fold. Because of their bulk, they interfere with vocal fold vibration, causing a rough, hoarse voice. They are most often seen in aggressive voice users, but may also result from medical conditions such as myxedema or heavy smoking. Videostroboscopy is virtually diagnostic and no additional evaluation is required. Polyps are managed surgically, and excision using microlaryngoscopy results in an improved voice

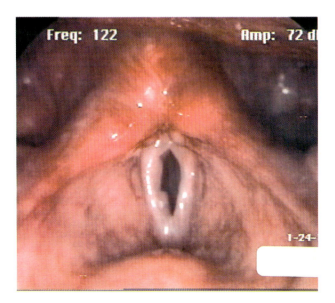

Figure 110 Polypoid degeneration is an asymmetrical polypoid change of the vocal fold mucosa diagnosed by videostroboscopy. Acute and chronic forms are recognized. The acute form develops in association with a chronic cough, such as in a long-standing upper respiratory infection, and, as the underlying illness and cough resolve, so too does the polypoid degeneration. Chronic polypoid degeneration, visually indistinguishable from the acute form, is associated with vocal abuse, gastrolaryngeal reflux and smoking. Complete evaluation occasionally involves laryngeal biopsy to exclude laryngeal carcinoma and papilloma. Management, as no surgical cure is available, involves correction of the underlying conditions, namely, elimination of patterns of vocal abuse, control of gastrolaryngeal reflux and cessation of smoking. Patients with the chronic form of polypoid degeneration may never regain a normal voice

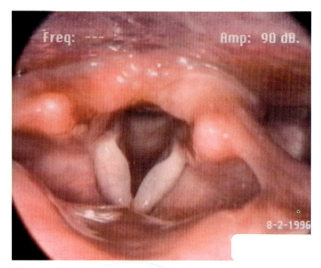

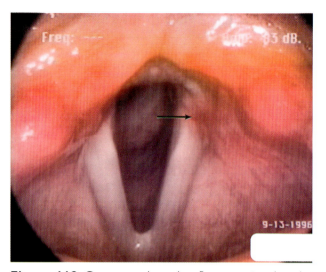

Figure 111 Reinke's edema, a common cause of chronic hoarseness, is associated with vocal abuse, smoking, chronic cough and gastrolaryngeal reflux. Reinke's edema, considered by some laryngologists to be part of the continuum of polypoid degeneration, differs from the latter in that both vocal folds are always symmetrically involved. With diagnostic videostroboscopy, the vocal folds have a sausage-like appearance due to accumulation of loose connective tissue, including mucopolysaccharides and water, within the superficial layer of the lamina propria. Patient evaluation is limited to assessment of underlying conditions, although laryngeal biopsy may be necessary to eliminate suspicion of laryngeal carcinoma. Management includes treatment of any associated aggravating factors. If patients do not respond to conservative management, surgical management involving removal of the excess loose connective tissue may be recommended. Rarely, the vocal folds become so enlarged that tracheotomy is required to maintain the airways

Figure 112 Gastroesophageal reflux may involve the laryngopharynx and result in a wide variety of laryngeal and pharyngeal symptoms, such as a burning sensation in the pharynx, a foreign-body sensation and chronic hoarseness. Examination findings include a generalized erythema of the larynx and pharynx, the posterior regions (arrowed) of which are the most susceptible. Interarytenoid erythema and edema are frequently present. Further evaluation includes a modified barium swallow and 24-h double-probe pH testing. Dietary modification and medical therapy are the mainstay of management, including modification of types of food and timing of meals. Fatty foods, large amounts of caffeinated beverages, alcohol, mint and chocolate should be avoided as should food intake less that 2 h before bedtime. Medical therapy includes antacids, H_2-receptor blockers and proton pump blockers

Figure 113 Gastrolaryngeal reflux and vocal abuse may cause ulcerations and, on occasions, granuloma formation on the body of the arytenoid cartilage. They may be either unilateral or bilateral. Most patients complain of posterolateral pharyngeal pain although, if the granulomas have a mucosal cover, they may be asymptomatic. Treatment involves management of gastrolaryngeal reflux, elimination of voice abuse and microlaryngeal excision. Lesions may recur as successful surgery depends on surgical wound healing without continued ulceration and granulation tissue formation

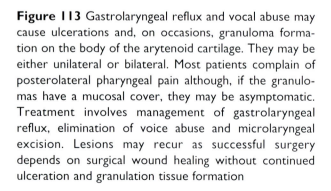

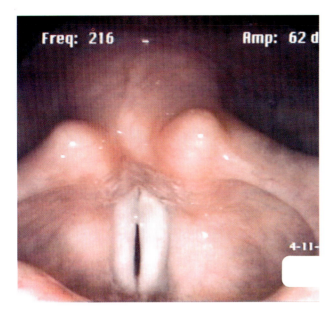

Figure 114 Patients in the eighth decade of life note changes in voice quality, strength and endurance which are associated with bowed vocal folds, as visualized on videostroboscopy. These changes are believed to be the result of atrophy of the thyroarytenoid muscle bulk due to aging. During sustained phonation, the vocal folds have a linear gap during the most closed phase of vocal fold vibration. Speech therapy may be helpful, but significant benefit is only derived by increasing the degree of medialization of the vocal folds either by injection of collagen into the thyroarytenoid muscle or by bilateral thyroplasty

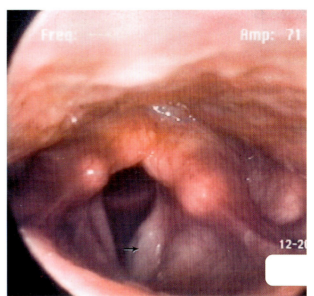

Figure 115 Patients with hoarseness lasting > 6 weeks should undergo a thorough laryngeal examination to ensure that squamous cell carcinoma of the larynx is not present. Laryngeal carcinoma (arrowed) is often associated with smoking and alcohol abuse. Fortunately, the vibratory edge of the vocal fold is most commonly involved and, thus, hoarseness presents early in the course of disease when the cure rate is high. Further evaluation includes a thorough head and neck examination and biopsy. For more advanced lesions, CT or MRI may help to delineate tumor extension. Treatment of small vocal fold carcinomas with either radiation therapy or surgical excision has a 90–95% chance of cure

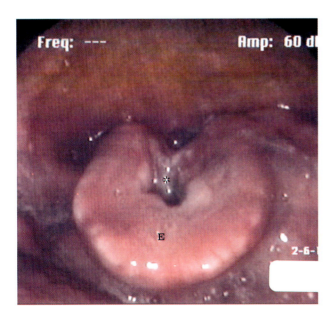

Figure 116 Advanced glottic squamous cell carcinoma is usually associated with long-standing hoarseness. Thorough examination of the larynx usually reveals disease involving both vocal folds and even vocal fold paralysis. (In the case shown here, the vocal folds, which should be visible at *, are not distinguishable.) Smoking and alcohol abuse are risk factors for the development of laryngeal carcinoma. CT or MRI is required to assess transcartilaginous spread; patients should also be evaluated for a second primary, such as bronchogenic or esophageal carcinoma. Therapy varies with the extent of disease, and may involve surgery, radiation therapy and/or chemotherapy. On occasion, airway obstruction by a large glottic carcinoma may precipitate emergency tracheotomy. E, epiglottis

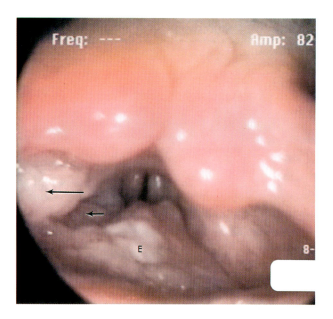

Figure 117 The second most common site for laryngeal carcinoma is the supraglottis (arrowed), especially the lingual surface of the epiglottis (E). In the case shown here, the vocal folds are normal. As with glottic carcinoma, smoking and alcohol abuse are recognized risk factors. Often, cervical lymphadenopathy is the presenting sign, and associated anterior pharyngeal or posterior lingual pain may be present. Growing silently, these cancers escape detection until late in their course. Evaluation involves either CT or MRI of the neck as well as biopsy. Management comprises either surgery or chemotherapy with radiation therapy

Index